HYDROGEN-OXYGEN INHALATION FOR TREATMENT OF

COVID-19

With Commentary from Zhong Nanshan

Other Related Titles from World Scientific

Combating a Crisis: The Psychology of Singapore's Response to COVID-19
by David Chan
ISBN: 978-981-122-055-5

The COVID-19 Epidemic in China
by Lawrence J Lau and Yanyan Xiong
ISBN: 978-981-122-250-4
ISBN: 978-981-122-419-5 (pbk)

COVID-19 from Traditional Chinese Medicine Perspective: Severe Clinical Cases in the Context of Syndrome Differentiation
by Luqi Huang, Hao Li, Wensheng Qi, Zhixu Yang and Qing Miao
ISBN: 978-981-122-874-2

COVID-19: From Basics to Clinical Practice
by Wenhong Zhang
ISBN: 978-981-122-206-1

Emergency Hospitals for COVID-19: Construction and Operation Manual
editor-in-chief Zhi Yan
translated by Ge Yan
ISBN: 978-981-122-302-0
ISBN: 978-981-122-303-7 (pbk)

Traditional Chinese and Western Medicine for Diagnosis and Treatment of Coronavirus Disease 2019 (COVID-19)
edited by Boli Zhang and Qingquan Liu
ISBN: 978-981-122-805-6

HYDROGEN-OXYGEN INHALATION FOR TREATMENT OF COVID-19

With Commentary from Zhong Nanshan

Kecheng Xu

Jinan University, China

World Scientific

EW JERSEY · LONDON · SINGAPORE · BEIJING · SHANGHAI · HONG KONG · TAIPEI · CHENNAI · TOKYO

Published by

World Scientific Publishing Co. Pte. Ltd.

5 Toh Tuck Link, Singapore 596224

USA office: 27 Warren Street, Suite 401-402, Hackensack, NJ 07601

UK office: 57 Shelton Street, Covent Garden, London WC2H 9HE

Library of Congress Cataloging-in-Publication Data

Names: Xu, Kecheng, 1940–   author. | Nanshan, Zhong, writer of added commentary.
Title: Hydrogen-oxygen inhalation for treatment of COVID-19 : with commentary from
    Zhong Nanshan / Kecheng Xu.
Description: New Jersey : World Scientific, [2020] | Includes bibliographical references and index.
Identifiers: LCCN 2020026842 | ISBN 9789811223297 (hardcover) |
    ISBN 9789811223303 (ebook for institutions) | ISBN 9789811223310 (ebook for individuals)
Subjects: MESH: Coronavirus Infections--therapy | Hydrogen--therapeutic use |
    Oxygen Inhalation Therapy | Pneumonia, Viral--therapy | Betacoronavirus
Classification: LCC RA644.C67 | NLM WC 505 | DDC 616.2/414--dc23
LC record available at https://lccn.loc.gov/2020026842

British Library Cataloguing-in-Publication Data
A catalogue record for this book is available from the British Library.

For any available supplementary material, please visit
https://www.worldscientific.com/worldscibooks/10.1142/11910#t=suppl

Typeset by Stallion Press
Email: enquiries@stallionpress.com

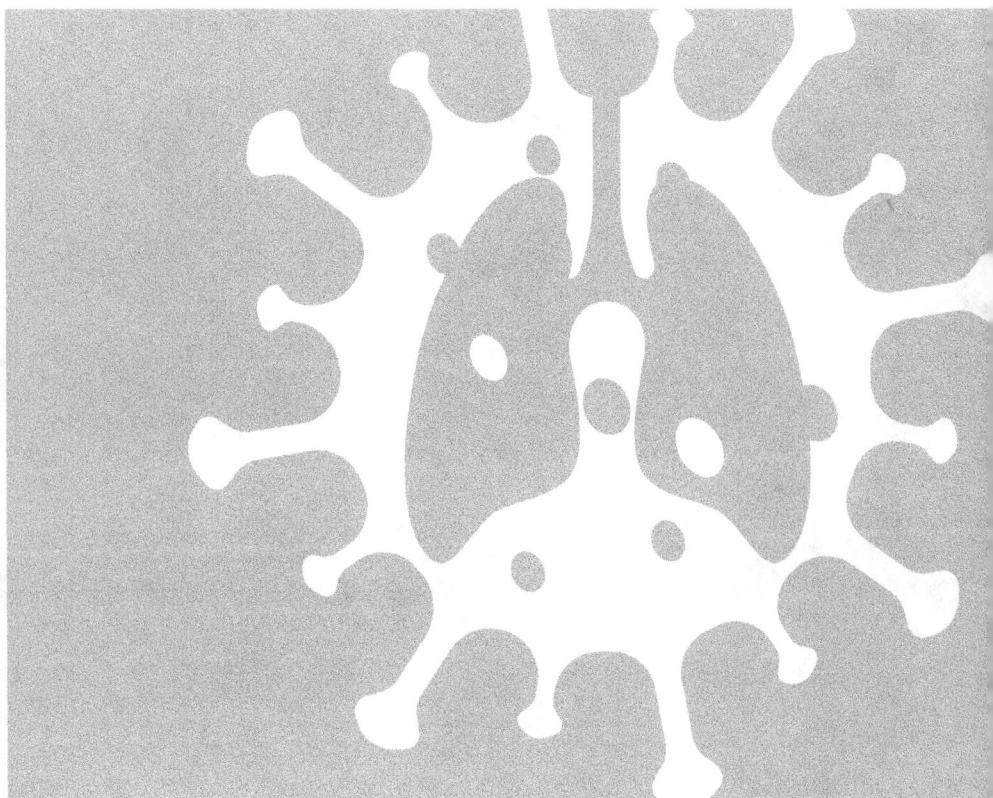

About the Authors

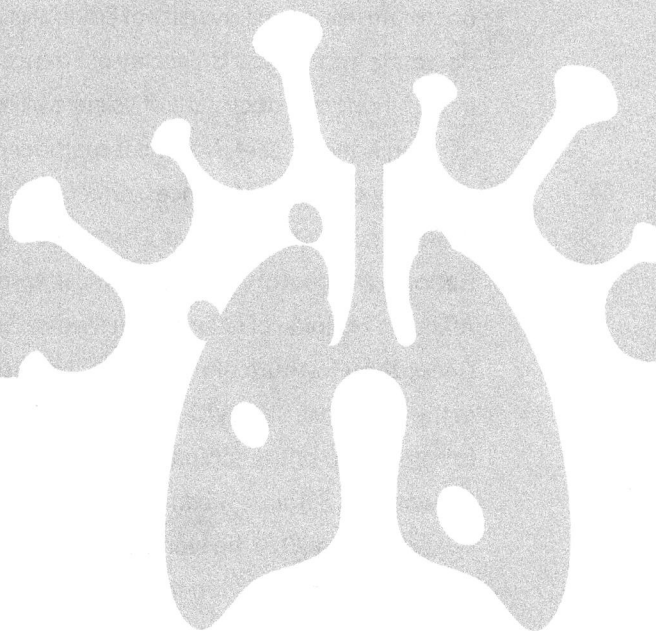

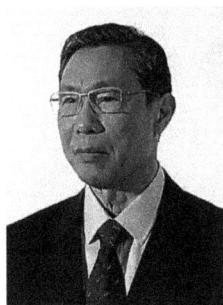

Zhong Nanshan, born in Nanjing, Jiangsu, China in 1936, is a professor, chief physician, doctoral supervisor, and academician of the Chinese Academy of Engineering. Since graduating from Beijing Medical College (now Peking University School of Medicine) in 1960, he has long been engaged in the medical treatment, teaching, and research of respiratory diseases, focusing on asthma, chronic obstructive pulmonary disease, respiratory failure and respiratory epidemic diseases. In recent years, he took the lead in introducing hydrogen-oxygen inhalation into the treatment of respiratory diseases and was the pioneer of *Clinical Hydrogen Medicine*. He received an honorary doctorate from the University of Edinburgh UK in 2007, an honorary doctorate from Macau University of Science and Technology in 2010, and an honorary doctorate of science from the Chinese University of Hong Kong in 2014. Now he is member of the Faculty of Chinese Academy of Medical Sciences, director of the State Key Laboratory of Respiratory Diseases of China (Guangzhou), director of the National Respiratory Disease Clinical Research Center of the First Affiliated Hospital of Guangzhou Medical University, director of the Guangzhou Institute of Respiratory Diseases, and a leading expert in the fight against COVID-19 in China , the leader of the High-Level Expert Group of the (China) National Health Commission. In 2004, he won the *Bethune Medal*, the highest honor of China's health system, and in 2020, he won the China *Medal of the Republic* for his outstanding contribution to the fight against COVID-19.

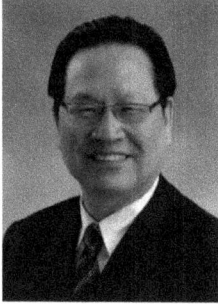

Xu Kecheng, born in Nantong, Jiangsu, China in 1940, is a professor, chief physician, and doctoral supervisor. He graduated from Nantong Medical College (now Nantong University School of Medicine) in 1963, studied liver cancer pathology and liver disease enzymology at Chiba University, Japan as a visiting professor in 1987, and worked as a visiting scholar at Wright State University, Ohio, USA in 1991 to study the pathology of *"small liver cancer"*. He has long been engaged in the clinical, teaching and research of gastrointestinal and liver diseases, especially in the minimally invasive treatment of solid tumors. He is a leading expert in cryosurgery and cryoablation of cancer in China and the world. In recent years, he has focused on cancer rehabilitation, taking the lead in introducing hydrogen medicine into cancer rehabilitation, and is the pioneer of *Clinical Hydrogen Oncology*. He is currently the honorary general dean of the Fuda Cancer Hospital affiliated to Jinan University, China the life honorary dean of the Institute of Biomedical Translational Research of Jinan University, and the director of Guangzhou Fuda Cancer Institute. He used to be the chairman of the International Society of Cryosurgery, and is currently the honorary chairman of the Asian Society of Cryosurgery and the chairman of the International Society of Clinical Hydrogen Medicine. He edited more than 20 monographs including *Modern Treament for Digestive Diseases* (Chinese), *Modern Cryosurgery for Cancer, Hydrogen Cancer Control* (Chinese). In 2012, he was awarded the *Bethune Medal*, the highest honor of China's health system. In 2013, he was awarded the title of *Model of the Times* in China, commending him for outstanding contributions in helping cancer patients.

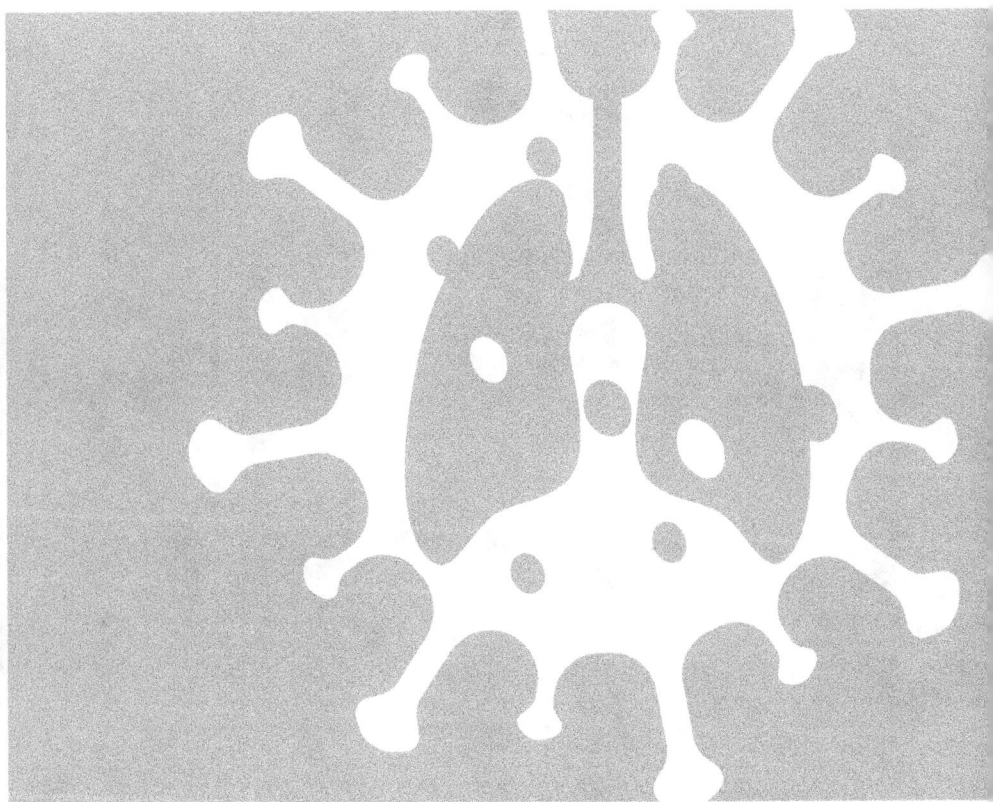

Preface

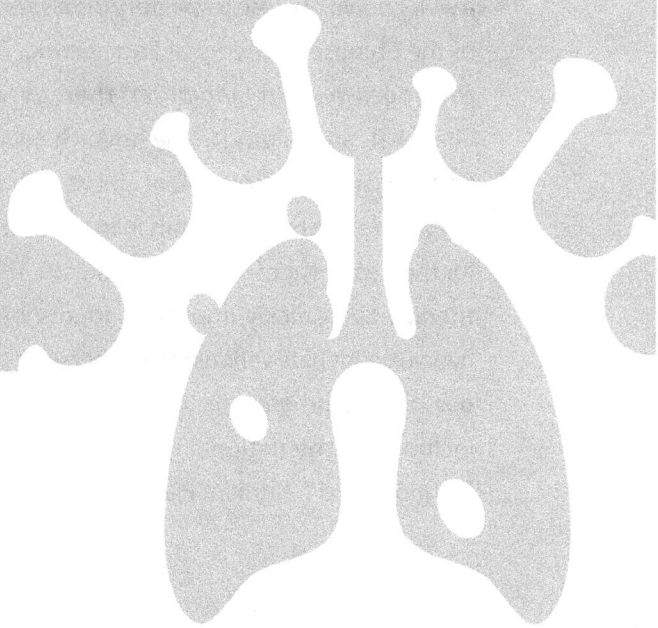

The coronavirus disease 2019 (COVID-19, caused by the virus SARS-CoV-2) is spreading all over the world, and human beings are facing this unprecedented disaster and crisis. In the face of serious threats to human lives, medicine seems a little helpless, because we have yet to obtain special drugs to fight against this new virus in the short term. But human beings have always been strong. Guided by the lofty goal of "let patients survive", countless medical workers have stepped forward without regard to their own mortality, reflecting the self-sacrificing qualities of doctors and the sacredness of medicine.

In the past few months of the fight against the COVID-19, the Chinese people have suffered tremendously, but have also endured trials, increased knowledge, and accumulated experience. To help COVID-19 patients suffering from dyspnea, Professor Zhong Nanshan, a well-known Chinese respiratory disease expert and an academician of the Chinese Academy of Engineering, first proposed the use of *"hydrogen-oxygen inhalation"* therapy. A Chinese company in Shanghai, specializing in the research and production of hydrogen and oxygen health equipment, donated thousands of *"hydrogen and oxygen atomizers"* to hospitals in Hubei and other affected provinces for the treatment of numerous patients. The results proved that the therapy can quickly improve patients' breathing difficulties and hypoxia, eliminate various respiratory symptoms, and may reduce the possibility of progression to severe disease. At present, the therapy is included in the national guidelines for China — the "COVID-19 Diagnosis and Treatment Plan (Trial Version 7)".

There is no life without oxygen. This is common knowledge. Hydrogen, the smallest molecule in nature, was not recognized for its potential medical value until the beginning of this century. Since then, it has quickly attracted worldwide attention to form a brand new discipline — *"Hydrogen Biology."* Since 2014, Academician Zhong Nanshan and his team have led the way in introducing hydrogen into clinical trials, pioneering *"Clinical Hydrogen Medicine".* A multi-center, randomized, and controlled study led by Academician Zhong Nanshan showed that inhalation of hydrogen-oxygen mixed gas for respiratory diseases, such as acute exacerbation of chronic obstructive pulmonary disease, can effectively reduce airway resistance, increase oxygen exchange and improve symptoms and respiratory function. In this fight against the COVID-19, Chinese medical workers have completed a multi-center, randomized, and controlled clinical trial of hydrogen-oxygen inhalation to treat COVID-19 pneumonia. The results are very encouraging.

Hydrogen is produced in the human colon all the time, and is considered to be *"physiological gas".* The hydrogen-oxygen mixed gas inhaled during treatment is generated from water electrolysis, so this treatment has great safety. The inhalation method is very simple and has great maneuverability, so it is suitable for almost all medical places, even in patients' homes.

It is undoubtedly of great practical significance to promote this simple, safe, and effective hydrogen-oxygen inhalation therapy to the world, so that people who are suffering from COVID-19 infection can benefit from it as soon as possible. To this end, we have written this book.

The book has 7 chapters in total. Chapter 1 reviews the biological effects of hydrogen, focusing on its antioxidant, anti-inflammatory, and cytoprotective effects and their molecular mechanism. Chapter 2 reviews the experimental research on hydrogen treatment of respiratory diseases, focusing on the principle of hyperoxic toxicity and mechanical ventilation-induced acute lung injury, and the improvement effect of hydrogen for them. Chapter 3 discusses the pathogenesis of human coronaviruses (HCoVs) infectious lung injury. Chapter 4 focuses on the relationship between respiratory virus infection and oxidant stress and reactive oxygen species (ROS). Chapters 3 and 4 lay the foundation for the subsequent introduction of hydrogen treatment. Chapter 5 introduces the clinical treatment of hydrogen for respiratory diseases. Chapter 6 discusses the rationality of the treatment of the COVID-19 pneumonia by hydrogen-oxygen inhalation based on the biological functions of hydrogen and the pathophysiological mechanism of the infection of HCoVs, especially the COVID-19. The last chapter introduces a real world evidence survey and a multi-center and controlled trial on hydrogen-oxygen inhalation for treatment of COVID-19 pneumonia, and proposes the principles and indications of this treatment.

COVID-19 is a new type of disease, and there are few literatures on this disease that can be referred to. This book mainly refers to the research results of other HCoVs, especially SARS and MERS CoV, in explaining the pathogenesis of the disease and the possible therapeutic effects of hydrogen.

Thanks very much to Academician Dr Zhong Nanshan. As a senior medical scientist, he made outstanding contributions to China's victory over SARS in 2003. At the critical moment when COVID-19 began to erupt in China, it was him who resolutely and decisively put forward the *"human-to-human"* argument, making great contributions to the fight against the pandemic in China and the world. A few years ago, under the influence and inspiration of Academician Zhong, I started research on hydrogen medicine and introduced hydrogen into the rehabilitation of cancer patients. The reason why I am the author of this book is actually because I am inspired by Academician Zhong's spirit of respecting science and attitude of fearless innovation. Academician Zhong reviewed the first draft of this book despite his busy schedule and also wrote a Commentary, all of which made me very grateful.

A huge thank you to the doctors and nurses who work in the frontline against the COVID-19 in China. They have provided this treatment to patients in extremely busy medical activities and conducted clinical research to obtain very valuable clinical application data and case information.

I sincerely thank Mr Jaiden Xu for correcting and polishing the text of this book, and would also like to thank Ms Ninnin Liu and Mrs Jinhua Wu for the creating the beautiful illustrations in this book.

In awe of life, as life is paramount. The ancient Chinese philosopher Lao Zi had a famous saying: "Greatness in simplicity".

Although hydrogen-oxygen inhalation therapy is "simple", but it can protect life, this is the "greatness". I hope the publication of this book will benefit patients, and provide inspiration and help to relevant clinicians and professional researchers.

This book is written within the shortest time possible. There are certainly many omissions and mistakes. Experts, colleagues, and readers are encouraged to criticize and correct.

Kecheng Xu, MD
May 6, 2020

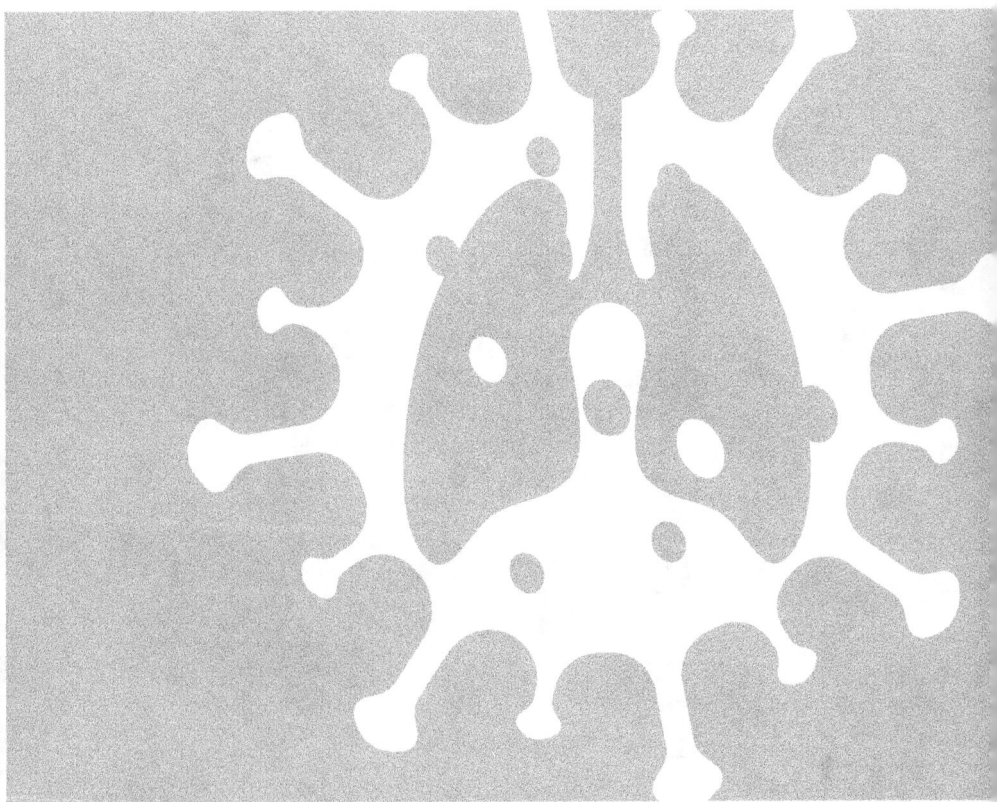

Commentary

By Zhong Nanshan, MD

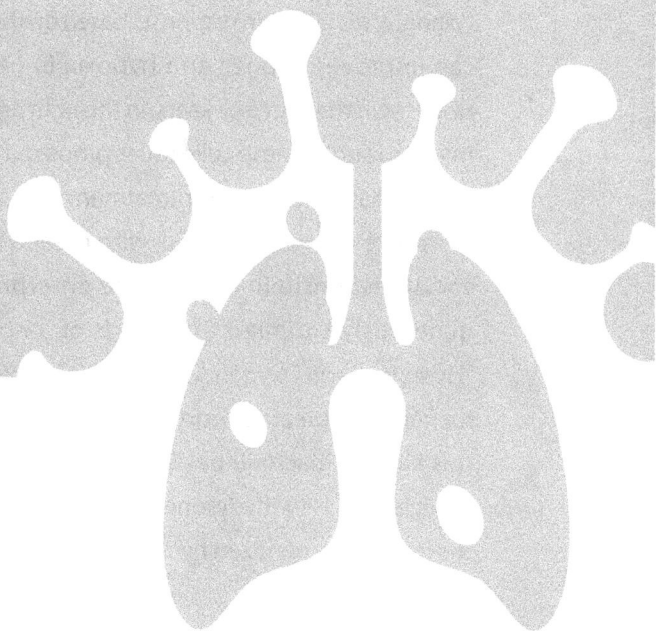

The Rationality and Feasibility of Hydrogen and Oxygen Inhalation as an Adjuvant Treatment of COVID-19

The coronavirus disease 2019 (COVID-19) pandemic is bringing huge disasters to mankind with its relentless worldwide dissemination and high morbidity and mortality [Harapan, *et al.*, 2020]. As there is no special antiviral drug that can be used at present, symptomatic management and maintenance of vital functions, improvement of symptoms, especially relief of dyspnea and correction of hypoxemia, have become the first tasks in clinical treatment. The scientific response to the crisis has been extraordinary, with a large number of COVID-19 trials emerging in an attempt to rapidly discover the pathogenesis of COVID-19 and potential therapeutic strategies [Wang, *et al.*, 2020]. In response, based on the research that hydrogen can improve dyspnea and hypoxia in patients with respiratory diseases in the past few years, in the fight against COVID-19 in China, my team and Chinese colleagues proposed use of "mixed hydrogen-oxygen gas inhalation" for treatment of COVID-19.

Since February of 2020, with great dedication and a sense of social responsibility, a Chinese enterprise from Shanghai has generously supplied thousands of a novel medical apparatus "Hydrogen and Oxygen Atomizers" (AMS-H-03) to the epidemic area for free. With great support from doctors and nurses of the frontline, this kind of machine has been used to treat COVID-19 patients, especially those with dyspnea, with good results. At present, in China, the inhalation of mixed hydrogen and oxygen gas has been written into the *National COVID-19 Diagnosis and Treatment Plan* (7th Edition) as a treatment method, and has been included as one of the adjuvant treatments for severe COVID-19.

As early as 300 BC, Chinese philosophers put forward the concept of "the harmony between man and nature" and advocated human life being in a high level of correspondence with nature. Among the gases that are critical to human life in nature, oxygen has long been one of the main methods of clinical first aid; although hydrogen has long been used in balloons and industrial fuels, its biological effects have long been ignored. In the 1970s, American scholars used a mixture of high-pressure hydrogen and oxygen to successfully treat experimental skin cancer [Dole, *et al.*, 1975]. At the beginning of this century, French scholars discovered that hydrogen can inhibit liver fibrosis [Gharib, *et al.*, 2001]. But none of these studies attracted attention. It was not until 2007 that Japanese scholars reported that inhalation of hydrogen gas can effectively improve the cerebral ischemic/reperfusion injury of experimental animals, and proposed that hydrogen molecules can selectively resist oxidation [Ohsawa, *et al.*, 2007]. This attracted worldwide attention. Chinese scholars first reported the therapeutic effect of hydrogen on neonatal hypoxic-ischemic mouse models in 2009 [Cai, *et al.*, 2009]. So far, there have been more than 1300 research papers on hydrogen biology.

The team of the First Affiliated Hospital of Guangzhou Medical University and the State Key Laboratory of Respiratory Disease where I work performed a clinical study of hydrogen and oxygen inhalation to treat airway stenosis, and found that hydrogen can effectively reduce the resistance of trachial stenosis and reduce the patient's inspiratory effort [Zhou, *et al.*, 2018]. Given that chronic obstructive pulmonary disease (COPD) is the most common respiratory system disease, we first observed the effects of inhalation of hydrogen and oxygen on improving respiratory function and inflammation in a mouse model of COPD induced by cigarette smoke [Liu, *et al.*, 2017]. This was followed by the organization of 10 hospitals in China carrying out randomized double-blind controlled studies on the treatment of acute exacerbations of COPD. The results showed that inhalation of a mixture of hydrogen and oxygen is better than simple oxygen inhalation in improving symptoms such as dyspnea and hypoxemia.

A large number of studies have confirmed that the therapeutic effects of hydrogen on diseases mainly lie in antioxidative, anti-inflammatory, and anti-apoptosis effects, as well as its protection on mitochondria and the endoplasmic reticulum, regulation of intracellular signaling pathways, and balancing of the immune cell subtypes [Iida, *et al.*, 2016; Tao, *et al.*, 2019]. Our findings demonstrated that hydrogen gas inhalation enhanced alveolar macrophage phagocytosis, which may be associated with the antioxidant effects of hydrogen gas and the activation of the Nrf2 pathway [Huang, *et al.*, 2019]. For respiratory diseases, hydrogen has a special role. According to Graham's law, the gas diffusion rate is inversely proportional to the square root of the density. The ratio of hydrogen to oxygen in the mixed gas we use is 2:1, and its molecular weight is much smaller than that of air and pure oxygen. Compared with air, the hydrogen-oxygen mixture has a lower density and a faster diffusion rate [Glauser, *et al.*, 1969], which makes it easier for oxygen to enter the alveoli and improves oxygen saturation. The mechanism of the aforementioned hydrogen-oxygen mixture to improve airway resistance largely depends on this.

The lung lesions of COVID-19 are closely related to the inflammatory storm triggered by the virus, and inflammation and oxidative stress promote each other [Harapan, *et al.*, 2020]. Pathologically, COVID-19 is mainly manifested as inflammation and exudation in the lower airways, including bronchi and alveoli [Wang, *et al.*, 2020]. Further studies have shown that several key biological processes, including reactive oxygen species (ROS), play crucial biological roles in inflammation [Lu, 2020]. This suggests that the application of hydrogen and oxygen inhalation to treat this disease is theoretically reasonable. In practice, according to clinical reports from many hospitals in China in the past six months, almost all patients felt reduced coughing and improved shortness of breath after inhaling a mixture of hydrogen and oxygen for a few hours, and chest pain and chest tightness were relieved one to two days later. From March to May 2020, the First Affiliated Hospital of Guangzhou Medical University, in conjunction with 11 hospitals in Shanghai, Hubei, Guangdong, Heilongjiang and other provinces and cities, conducted a *real-world* survey on the effectiveness of hydrogen and oxygen inhalation in the treatment of COVID-19, and the results confirmed that this simple and easy method can quickly improve respiratory symptoms, relieve dyspnea, improve hypoxia, and reduce disease severity and progression [Guan, *et al.*, 2020].

Hydrogen gas is the lightest and smallest molecule in natural gas. Normal human intestinal bacteria produce 300-400 ml every day, so it is called "physiological gas" [Levitt, 1969, 1980]. Moreover, because of its relatively low reducibility, it can selectively neutralize "toxic" hydroxyl ($\cdot$OH) and nitrosoperoxide (ONCO-) with no affection of the signal-like reactive oxygen species required for normal metabolism in the body, so it has a high degree of biological safety [Sano, *et al.*, 2017]. The current equipment used for hydrogen and oxygen inhalation therapy has been approved by the Chinese FDA as a Class III medical device, which provides extremely favorable conditions for long-term use of this therapy for patients, especially home applications.

Recently, there have been more and more reports on the extrapulmonary manifestations and complications of COVID-19 [Gupta, *et al.*, 2020]. The angiotensin-converting enzyme 2 (ACE2) receptor is the main mechanism by which the COVID-19 virus enters the cell. In addition to the lung, it is also expressed in many tissues outside the lung. The extensive damage of multiple organs in severe COVID-19 patients may be related to the expression of ACE2 [Vabret, *et al.*, 2020]. According to reports, as many as 40% of COVID-19 patients have various neurological symptoms, such as dizziness, ataxia, seizures, loss of taste and smell, vision defects, and even confusion; heart, kidney, and liver damage are also often occurs [Acharya, *et al.*,2020]. Timely prevention and treatment of these extrapulmonary symptoms and complications is an important part of COVID-19 treatment.

In addition, based on our past experience in the treatment of SARS, we must pay special attention to the possibility of pulmonary fibrosis complications in patients who survived COVID-19, especially severely ill patients. During lung virus infection, oxidative stress is elevated in epithelial cells, which stimulates the production and release of transforming growth factor-β (TGF-β), causing excessive migration, proliferation, activation of fibroblasts and myofibroblasts differentiation, leading to airway remodeling. On the other hand, TGF-β can promote the expression of collagen induced by angiotensin II (AngII). In addition, TGF-β can act on alveolar macrophages to stimulate the secretion of IL-4, IL-6 and IL-13, thereby promoting the development of fibrosis [Delpino and Quarleri, 2020]. In this case, activated fibroblasts further induced the damage and death of alveolar epithelial cells, thus forming a vicious circle of profibrotic epithelial cell-fibroblast interactions nourished by TGF-β leading to the formation of non-functional scar tissue (Li, *et al.*, 2016).

These considerations will help us reduce or prevent these complications, thereby speeding up the best clinical outcome. All these pathological damages are accompanied by excessive production of ROS and inflammation. As mentioned earlier, molecular hydrogen has been widely proven to be a selective antioxidant and anti-inflammatory agent. The currently available data indicate that hydrogen, especially when mixed with oxygen, can prevent and treat diseases or pathological states of various systems [Ono, *et al.*, 2017; Sano, *et al.*, 2017;Yan, *et al.*, 2019; Zhang, *et al.*, 2019; Camara, *et al.*, 2019] . It is reasonable to speculate that the inhalation of hydrogen and oxygen mixtures in COVID-19 patients, especially at home after discharge, is undoubtedly of significance for preventing and improving these complications. Clinical trials on this subject are currently underway.

In summary, for COVID-19, hydrogen and oxygen inhalation therapy is suitable for the following aims.

- To rapidly improve symptoms and shorten the length of hospitalization in the majority of patients showing mild symptoms;
- To be used as an adjuvant treatment in severe and critically ill patients;
- To prevent progression from mild to severe cases;
- To prevent or improve complications of COVID-19.

The World Health Organization claims that COVID-19 cannot be eliminated quickly. Therefore, it is of great significance to adopt simple, effective and safe methods to maintain the body's resistance to systemic diseases. Hydrogen and oxygen inhalation therapy is one of the methods worth promoting. The Chinese and people all over the world are a community with a shared future. In the current severe situation of COVID-19, it is our sacred responsibility for people from all over the world, especially those in the medical profession, to help and support each other, develop international cooperation, and share successful experiences. Therefore, I recommend this therapy to the world.

Professor Xu Kecheng, as a senior internal medicine expert, has devoted himself to researching clinical application of hydrogen medicine in recent years. Under the circumstance of the COVID-19 pandemic, out of mission and the commitment to healthcare, Professor Xu analyzed published literature at great length, combined his findings with Chinese clinical practice, and compiled "Hydrogen-Oxygen Inhalation for Treatment of COVID-19". I admire Professor Xu's outstanding work and express my great respect.

This book first introduces the biological effects of hydrogen and the role of oxidative stress in the pathogenesis of viral lung injury, as well as the experimental research and clinical practice of hydrogen in the treatment of various diseases, and then discusses the rationality of the application of hydrogen-oxygen inhalation therapy in COVID-19. Finally, the *real world survey* results of hydrogen and oxygen inhalation treatment for COVID-19 patients jointly conducted by many hospitals in China are introduced. This book not only introduces basic and experimental research, but also has clinical treatment data. It is a monograph combining theory and practice. The author cited hundreds of documents, reflecting the progress in the latest research. Here, I am honored to recommend it to readers.

Of course, COVID-19 is a new disease, and our understanding of it is still very superficial. The application of hydrogen and oxygen inhalation therapy is still in its infancy. There must be content in this book that needs to be revised and supplemented. But this will not damage the enthusiasm and passion of the author, nor will it belittle the extraordinary efforts made by the author in an extraordinary period. As an old friend of Professor Xu and commissioned by Professor Xu, I call on relevant experts, especially clinicians who are fighting COVID-19, to provide valuable comments and criticisms so that they can be revised in the reprint.

World Scientific Publishing Co. has released this book within the shortest time frame possible. This is a major contribution to the medical community's fight against COVID-19. As a fighter who is fighting COVID-19, I would like to express my gratitude.

I would like to take this opportunity to express my sincere gratitude to the frontline clinical experts and medical staff who have made great contributions in the clinical observation and trial of hydrogen and oxygen treatment of COVID-19.

References

1. Acharya A, Kevadiya BD, Gendelman HE, *et al.* (2020). SARS-CoV-2 infection leads to neurological dysfunction. *J Neuroimmune Pharmacol.* 15(2), pp. 167–173.

2. Cai J, Kang Z, Sun XJ,,*et al.* (2009). Neuroprotective effects of hydrogen saline in neonatal hypoxia-ischemia rat model. *Brain Res.* 1256, pp. 129–137.

3. Camara R, Matei N, Camara J, *et al.* (2019). Hydrogen gas therapy improves survival rate and neurological deficits in subarachnoid hemorrhage rats: a pilot study. *Med Gas Res.* 9(2), pp. 74–79.

4. Delpino MV and Quarleri I. (2020). SARS-CoV-2 pathogenesis: imbalance in the renin-angiotensin system favors lung fibrosis. *Front Cell Infect Microbiol.* 10, pp. 340.

5. Dole M, Wilson FR, Fife WP. (1975). Hyperbaric hydrogen therapy: a possible treatment for cancer. *Science.* 190(4210), pp. 152–154.

6. Gharib B, Hanna S, Abdallahi OM, *et al.* (2001). Anti-inflammatory properties of molecular hydrogen: investigation on parasite-induced liver inflammation. *C R Acad Sci III.* 324(8), pp. 719–724.

7. Glauser SC, Glauser EM, Rusy BF. (1969). Influence of gas density and viscosity on the work of breathing. *Arch Environ Health.* 19(5), pp. 654–660.

8. Guan WJ, Wei CH, Chen AL, *et al.* (2020). Hydrogen/oxygen mixed gas inhalation improves disease severity and dyspnea in patients with Coronavirus disease 2019 in a recent multicenter, open-label clinical trial. *J Thorac Dis.* 12(6), pp. 3448–3452.

9. Gupta A, Madhavan MV, Sehgal K, *et al.* (2020). Extrapulmonary manifestations of COVID-19. *Nat Med.* 26(7), pp. 1017–1032.

10. Harapan H, Itoh N, Yufika A, *et al.* (2020). Coronavirus disease 2019 (COVID-19): a literature review. *J Infect Public Health.* 13(5), pp. 667–673.

11. Huang P, Wei S, Huang W, *et al.* (2019). Hydrogen gas inhalation enhances alveolar macrophage phagocytosis in an ovalbumin-induced asthma model. *Int Immunopharmacol.* 74, pp. 105646.

12. Li C, Hancock MA, Sehgal P, *et al.* (2016). Soluble CD109 binds TGF-β and antagonizes TGF-β signalling and responses. *Biochem J.* 473(5), pp. 537–547.

13. Iida A, Nosaka N, Yumoto T, *et al.* (2016). The clinical application of hydrogen as a medical treatment. *Acta Med Okayama.* 70(5), pp. 331–337.

14. Levitt MD. (1969). Production and excretion of hydrogen gas in man. *N Engl J Med.* 281(3), pp. 122–127.

15. Levitt MD. (1980). Intestinal gas production--recent advances in flatology. *N Engl J Med*. 302(26), pp. 1474–1475.

16. Liu X, Ma C, Wang X, *et al.* (2017). Hydrogen coadministration slows the development of COPD-like lung disease in a cigarette smoke-induced rat model. *Int J Chron Obstruct Pulmon Dis*. 12, pp. 1309–1324.

17. Lu QB. (2020). Reaction cycles of halogen species in the immune defense: implications for human health and diseases and the pathology and treatment of COVID-19. *Cells*. 9(6), pp. 1461.

18. Ohsawa I, Ishikawa M, Takahashi K, *et al.* (2007). Hydrogen acts as a therapeutic antioxidant by selectively reducing cytotoxic oxygen radicals. *Nat Med*. 13(6), pp. 688–694.

19. Ono H, Nishijima Y, Ohta S, *et al.* (2017). Hydrogen gas inhalation treatment in cerebral infarction: a randomized controlled clinical study on safety and neuroprotection. *J Stroke Cerebrovasc Dis*. 26(11), pp. 2587–2594.

20. Sano M, Suzuki M, Homma K, *et al.* (2017). Promising novel therapy with hydrogen gas for emergency and critical care medicine. *Acute Med Surg*. 5(2), pp. 113–118.

21. Tao G, Song GH, Qin S.(2019).Molecular hydrogen: current knowledge on mechanism in alleviating free radical damage and diseases *Acta Biochim Biophys Sin (Shanghai)* 51(12),pp.1189–1197 .

22. Vabret N,Britton GJ, Gruber C,*et al.*(2020).Immunology of COVID-19: current state of the science. *Immunity*. 52(6),pp.910–941.

23. Wang J, Jiang M, Chen X, Montaner LJ. (2020). Cytokine storm and leukocyte changes in mild versus severe SARS-CoV-2 infection: review of 3939 COVID-19 patients in China and emerging pathogenesis and therapy concepts. *J Leukoc Biol*. 108(1), pp. 17–41.

24. Yan M, Yu Y, Mao X, *et al.*(2019).Hydrogen gas inhalation attenuates sepsis-induced liver injury in a FUNDC1-dependent manner. *Int Immunopharmacol.* 71, pp.61–67.

25. Zhang Y, Tan S, Xu J, Wang T.(2018).Hydrogen therapy in cardiovascular and metabolic Diseases: from bench to bedside. *Cell Physiol Biochem.* 47(1), pp.1–10.

26. Zhou ZQ, Zhong CH, Su ZQ, *et al.* (2018). Breathing hydrogen-oxygen mixture decreases inspiratory effort in patients with tracheal stenosis. *Clin Invest.* doi: 1159/ 000492031.

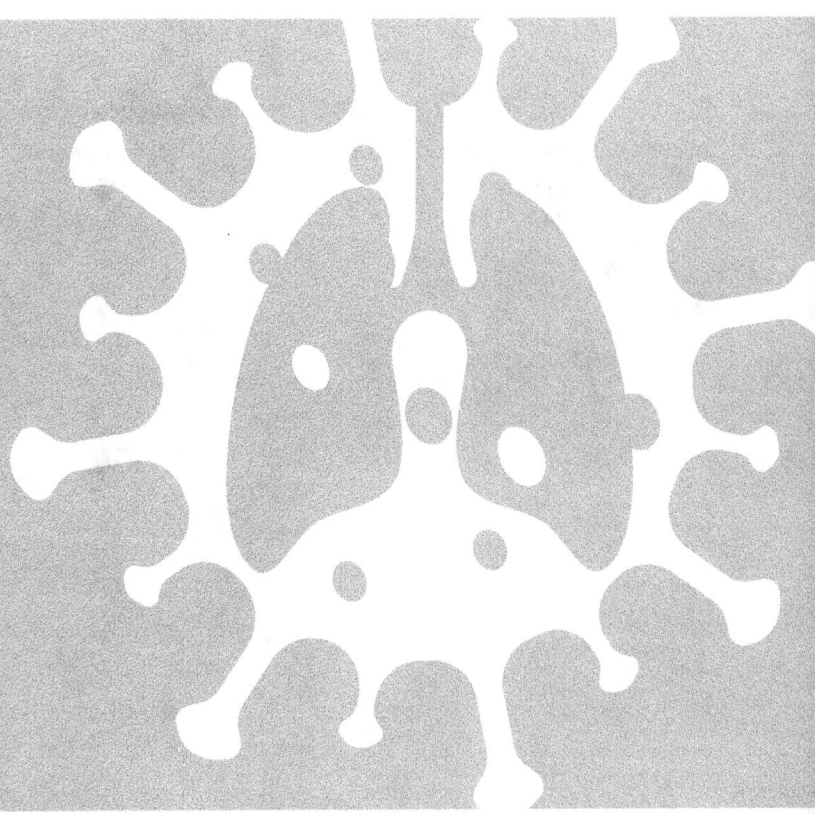

Contents

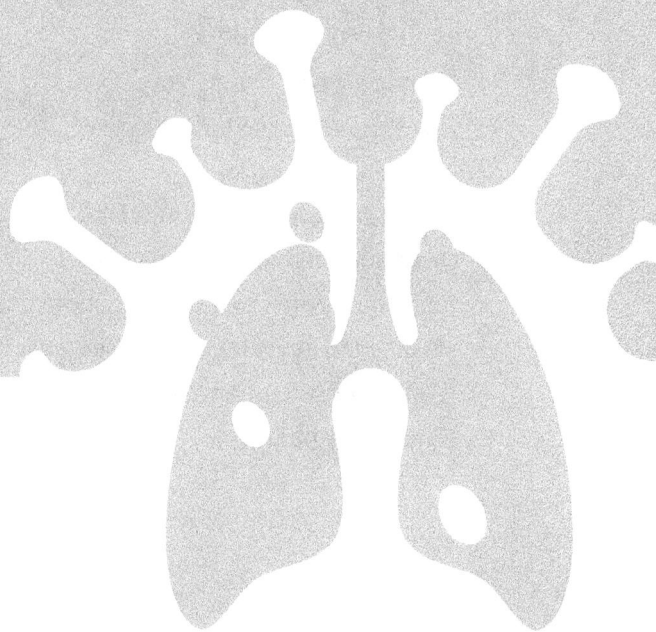

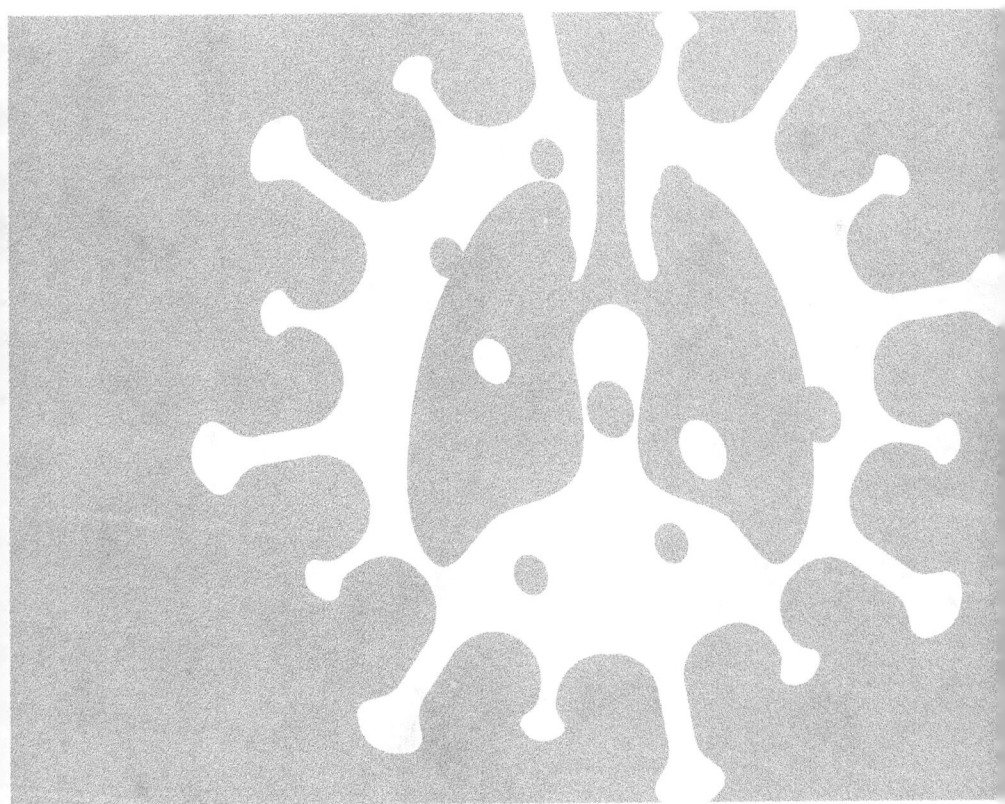

Introduction

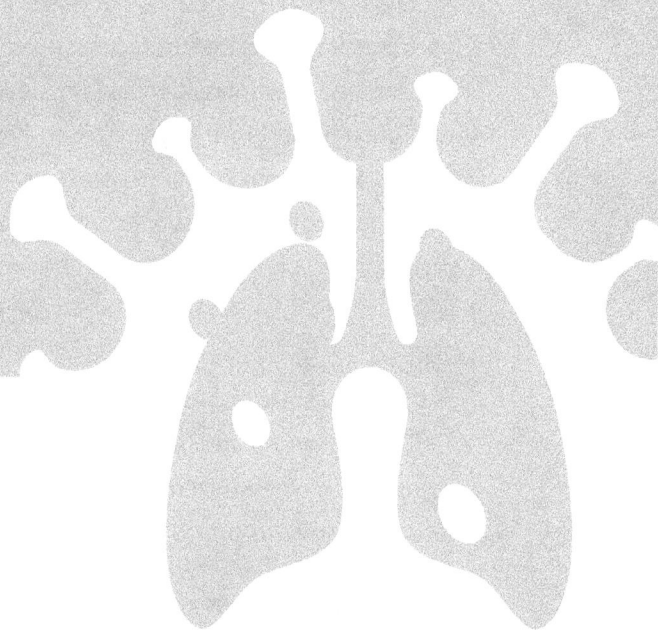

The coronavirus disease 2019 (COVID-19) has become a pandemic that is threatening the world. Although most patients have mild symptoms and good prognosis, some patients develop severe symptoms and die from multiple organ complications. Many uncertainties remain with regards to the pathogenesis of the virus infection in humans, including virus-host interaction and immune function against invasive pathogens. At the moment, there is no specific antiviral drug against the virus, while the therapeutic strategies to deal with the infection are only supportive.

China has achieved a decisive victory in the huge challenge to combat this new disease and has accumulated rich experience. In the absence of an established treatment plan, many options have been explored in the treatment of COVID-19. Some of these treatments may have been tried out of despair, but some of them show initial hope. China's practice shows that the focus of treatment should save critically ill patients and prevent mild cases from developing into severe ones. It is of great importance to comprehensively take various effective measures. Inhalation of a mixed gas consisting of 67% hydrogen and 33% oxygen, a seemingly simple but well-founded treatment that is primarily based on the biological properties of molecular hydrogen, has shown encouraging results in the comprehensive treatment of COVID-19.

In the recently published Chinese national guidelines — the "COVID-19 Diagnosis and Treatment Plan (Trial Version 7)", inhalation of hydrogen-oxygen mixed gas is used as a treatment measure to improve disease symptoms and respiratory function.

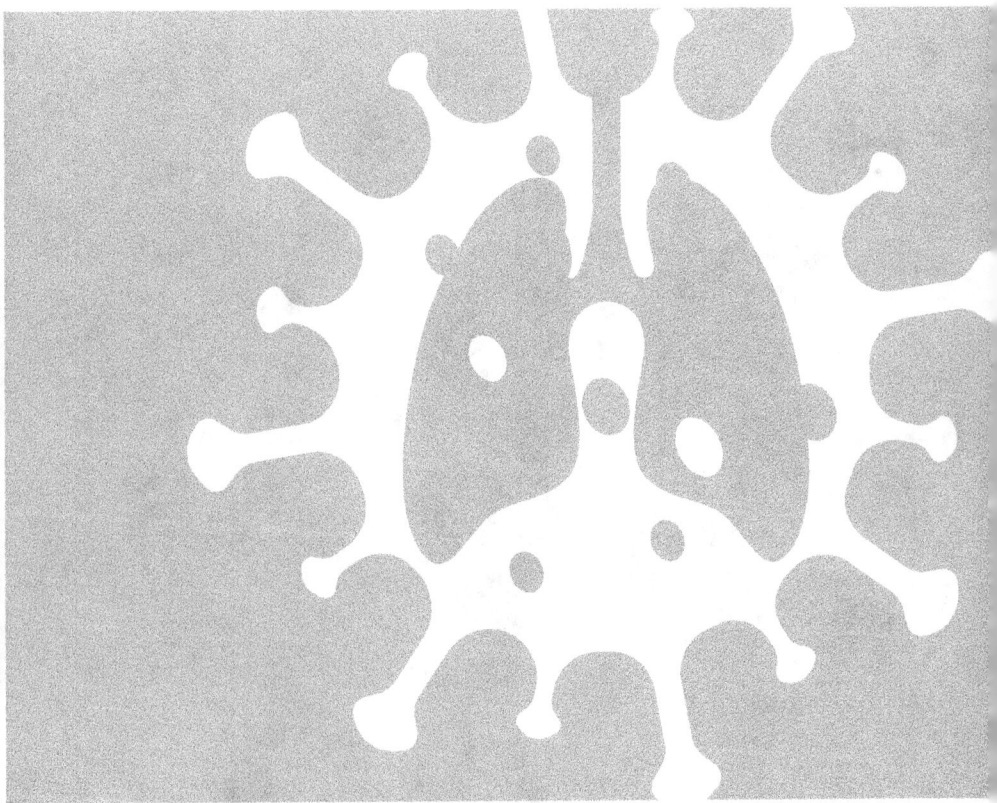

Hydrogen Gas and Its Biological Effects

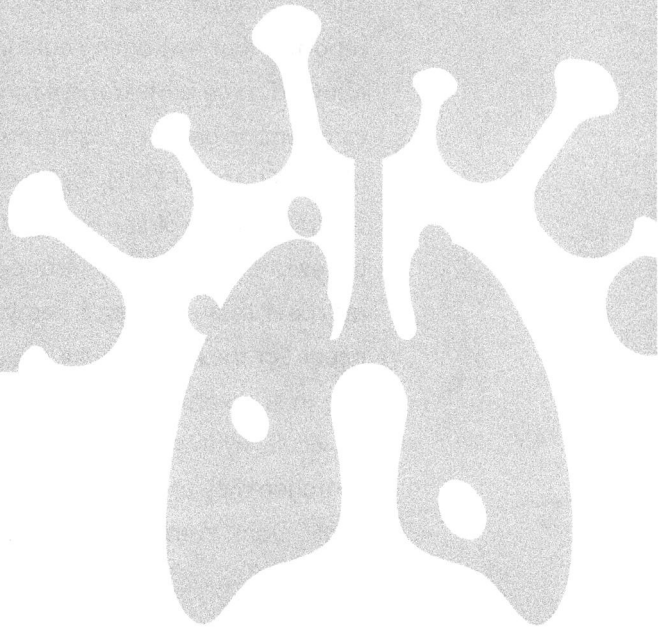

The hydrogen molecule (H_2), formed by two hydrogen atoms, is colorless, odorless, and the smallest and simplest molecule in nature. Most mammals, including humans, do not synthesize hydrogenase, which is a catalyst that activates H_2. Therefore, H_2 has long been considered as an inert gas in mammalian cells.

In the past two hundred years, three papers have proved that hydrogen is a therapeutic gas, and they are worth mentioning here.

- The first paper was published by Pilcher in 1888. They used hydrogen to blow into the gastrointestinal tract to locate visceral damage and avoid unnecessary surgery. However, this is using the physical properties of hydrogen without discovering its biological potential.

- The second paper was from Dole, *et al.* in 1975, who reported that hydrogen could inhibit cancer cells. They allowed mice with transplanted skin squamous cell carcinoma to breathe a high-pressure mixed gas consisting of 2.5% O_2 and 97.5% H_2 for 2 weeks. The surprising result was that tumor volume was greatly reduced. The authors believed that the mechanism behind this phenomenon may be H_2 catalyzed radical decay. This is a groundbreaking paper. For the first time, it is hypothesized that H_2 plays a role in scavenging •OH radicals, but perhaps because molecular hydrogen is too "simple", or the high-pressure hydrogen they used has technical difficulties in practical applications, even though their article is published in the famous magazine *Science*, it has not attracted the attention of academia and seems to be forgotten.

- In 2001, Gharib, *et al.* published the third article, which further reported the antioxidant effect of hydrogen in the body. They found that inhaled H_2 has a therapeutic effect on chronic hepatitis associated with schistosomiasis, and they believed that the anti-inflammatory effect of hydrogen may be due to its ability to scavenge hydroxyl radicals.

However, the above findings did not arouse people's attention until Ohsawa, *et al.* [2007] who demonstrated the selective antioxidant capacity and therapeutic effect of hydrogen on cerebral ischemia in 2007. This is a pioneering study which reported that H_2 can selectively reduce toxic free radicals such as hydroxyl radicals ($\bullet OH$) and peroxynitrite ($ONOO^-$) in cultured cells, but not other reactive species such as superoxide (O_2^-), hydrogen peroxide (H_2O_2), and nitric oxide ($NO\bullet$). Since then, the number of papers on hydrogen biology has increased dramatically [Ohsawa, *et al.*, 2007; Ge, *et al.*, 2017].

In the past 10 years or more, basic and clinical studies have shown that H_2 is an important biological regulator, which not only has the specific activity of scavenging hydroxyl radicals and peroxynitrite, but also has other properties such as reduction of inflammatory reactions, modulation of signal transduction, alteration of gene expressions, mitochondrial protection, and anti-apoptotic and immune-regulating effects on cells and organs (Figure 1-1).

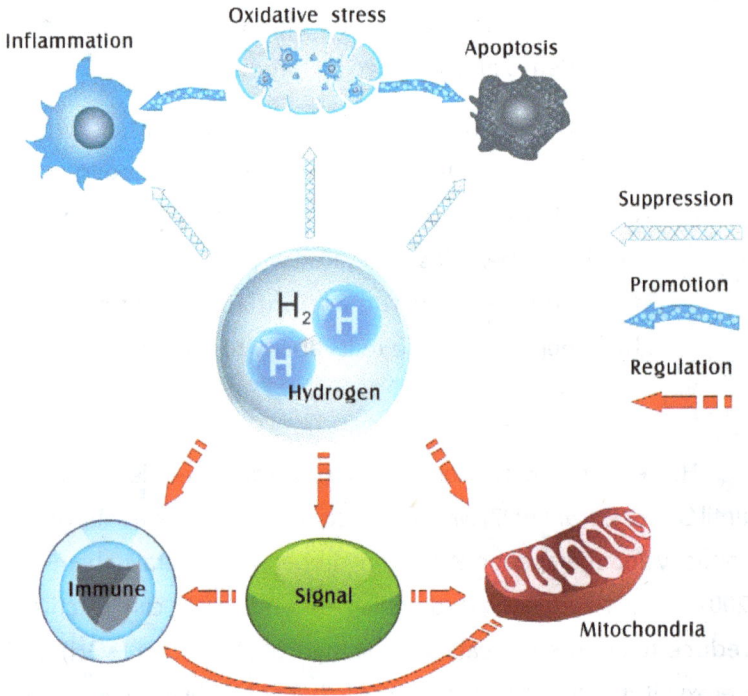

Figure 1-1 The biological effects of molecular hydrogen (H_2).

Anti-oxidant effect

The anti-oxidant effect of molecular hydrogen is focused on its specific scavenging activity of hydroxyl radicals ($\bullet OH$) and peroxynitrite ($ONOO-$) which induce oxidant stress.

Formation and cytotoxicity of reactive oxygen/nitrogen species

Reactive oxygen/reactive nitrogen species (ROS/RNS) is a redox by-product and occurs during normal cellular metabolism. Active oxygen is continuously produced during metabolism, and exists in the form of free radicals, ions and molecules with a single unpaired electron, and has high reactivity. Broadly, ROS is grouped as oxygen-free radicals which include hydroxyl radical ($\bullet$OH), superoxide (O_2^-), organic radicals (R$\bullet$), alkoxyl radicals (RO$\bullet$), nitric oxide (NO$\bullet$), peroxyl radicals (ROO$\bullet$), disulfides (RSSR), thiyl peroxyl radicals (RSOO$\bullet$), sulfonyl radicals (ROS$\bullet$), and thiyl radicals (RS$\bullet$). Other forms of ROS include singlet oxygen ($O\bullet_2$), hydrogen peroxide (H_2O_2), organic hydroperoxides (ROOH), ozone/trioxygen (O_3), hypochloride (HOCl), nitrosoperoxycarbonate anion (O=NOOCO$-$2), nitrocarbonate anion (O_2NOCO$-$2), peroxynitrite (ONCO$^-$), nitronium (NO^+2), dinitrogen dioxide (N_2O_2), and high-reacting lipid or carbohydrate derived including carbonyl compounds.

ROS is mainly produced from mitochondria. During cellular respiration, electrons are transported through a series of mitochondrial complexes to the terminal electron acceptor, the molecule oxygen (O_2). During cell metabolism, electrons released from the electron transport chain (ETC) react with O_2 to form superoxide (O_2^-) free radicals. Superoxide radicals generated at complexes I and III are released into the intermembrane space. The intermembrane space contains 80% of the superoxide radicals produced by the mitochondria, and the remaining 20% is produced by the mitochondrial matrix. Mitochondrial permeable transition pores in the outer membrane of mitochondria allow superoxide radicals to enter the cytoplasm and transform into hydrogen peroxide in the cytoplasm. Superoxide dismutase (via Cu/ZnSOD), located in the mitochondrial matrix (MnSOD) or cytoplasm, catalyzes the reaction. In addition, aquaporin 8 acts as a channel for the release of hydrogen peroxide from the cell membrane [Venditti and Di Meo, 2020].

Another important signaling associated with ROS production is the membrane-bound enzyme NADPH oxidases (Nox). However, the Nox-mediated release of ROS, by the mechanism of the oxidative burst, is commonly associated with the immune response and mediated by cells of the immune system, such as macrophages and neutrophils, and by inflammatory reactions. The Nox-mediated mechanism involves various stages such as activation of Nox genes and transmembrane proteins for the transport of electrons across biological membranes where there is a reduction of molecular oxygen into superoxide by Nox as a part of redox signaling [Lee and Paull, 2020].

There is another major site for the generation of ROS termed as peroxisomes where superoxide and H_2O_2 are generated through xanthine oxidase in the peroxisomal matrix and membranes.

Other sources of ROS include endogenous metabolites, such as fatty acids and prostaglandins, and exogenous ingredients, including drugs, flavors, colorants, antioxidants, and the like. These substances are processed in the smooth endoplasmic reticulum and converted into free radicals, especially •OH. Macrophages and white blood cells, as part of the immune response, contribute to the formation of free radicals.

In normal cells, ROS is involved in the regulation of signaling processes of cell division, immune regulation, autophagy, inflammation, and stress-related responses. However, if these oxidants, mainly •OH and ONOO-, are generated in an uncontrolled manner, they can cause oxidative stress, inducing cytotoxicity and cell function loss.

Reactive oxygen species-mediated oxidative stress induces alteration of cell membrane lipid bilayer by the process of lipid peroxidation of polyunsaturated fatty acids. This causes the generation of lipoperoxyl radical (LOO•), which, in turn, reacts with a lipid to yield a lipid-based radical and a lipid hydroperoxide (LOOH). These LOOHs are unstable, and they generate new peroxyl and alkoxy radicals and decompose to secondary products. Free radicals produced during lipid peroxidation have very minute and local effects because of their short life. However, the breakdown products of lipid peroxides, such as aldehydes, malondialdehyde, hexanal, and 4-hydroxynonenal (HNE), serve as "oxidative stress second messengers" due to their prolonged half-life and their ability to diffuse from their site of generation. Among the products of lipid peroxidation, HNE is chemically reactive because of its highly electrophilic nature and it easily reacts with glutathione, proteins, and DNA which leads to the covalent modifications on macromolecules [Sato, *et al.*, 2008; Kumari, *et al.*, 2018].

Oxidative stress activates multiple transcription factors, including nuclear factor (NF)-κB, activating protein 1, p53, hypoxia-inducible factor 1-α (HIF-1α), matrix metalloproteinases, peroxisome proliferator activation receptors-γ, β-catenin/Wnt, and nuclear factor erythroid 2-related factor 2 (Nrf2).

Acute and chronic excessive intracellular increases of ROS are implicated in the initiation and progression of many diseases. ROS is considered as a common factor of diseases induced by many

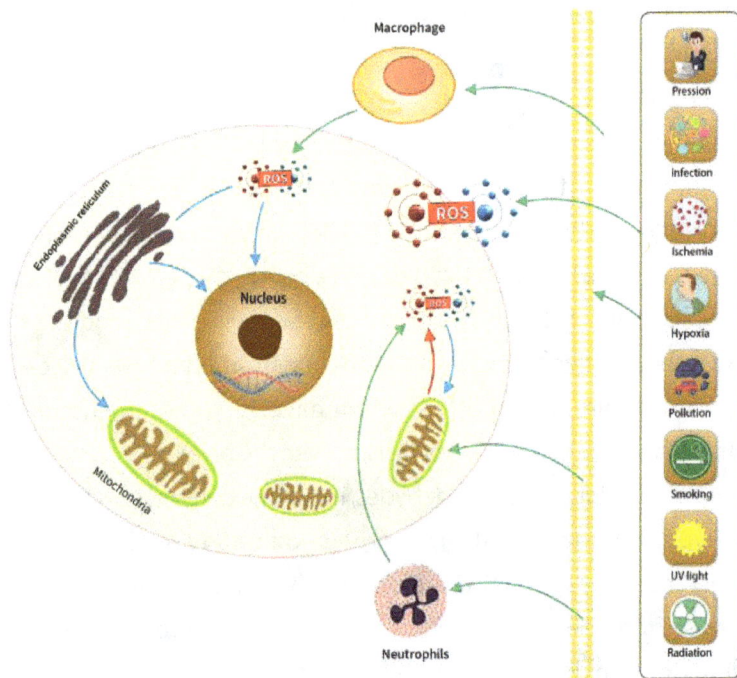

Figure 1-2 The formation of ROS induced by many factors and its effect on nucleus and mitochondria.

factors, such as hypoxia, ischemia, psychological pression, radiation, ultraviolet light, infection (virus), pollution, and smoking [Geto, *et al.*, 2020] (Figure 1-2).

Scavenging toxic ROS/RNS

As mentioned, ROS is the common key to the occurrence and progression of many diseases. Therefore, the removal of ROS is extremely important in the treatment and prevention of diseases.

However, conventional antioxidants have little effect in eliminating ROS. This is because not all of ROS is destructive, only •OH (hydroxyl radical) is a strong oxidant that causes tissue damage, and some beneficial free radicals such as superoxide and hydrogen peroxide can enhance endogenous antioxidant mechanisms through signal transduction pathways, thus playing an important role in body metabolism. Common potent antioxidants, such as vitamins C and E, indiscriminately eliminate both destructive and beneficial ROS, and therefore, excessive amounts of commonly used antioxidants are sometimes not only unhelpful to health, but harmful. Moreover, these antioxidants do not easily penetrate biofilms, that is, they cannot directly enter the cells to play a biological role.

Hydrogen is a weak reducing agent, and its redox reaction occurs only under strong oxidants [Sano, *et al.*, 2018]. Moreover, hydrogen has a low molecular weight and can quickly diffuse through cell membranes and lipid bilayers, reaching the nucleus and mitochondria where most aggressive ROS is located (Figure 1-3).

There is already a consensus that the hydrogen molecule represents an effective and non-toxic molecule with broad potential to mitigate/eliminate the negative effects of toxic ROS/RNS. It is speculated that, based on the exothermic reaction of $H_2 + •OH \rightarrow H_2O + H•$ followed by the $H• + O_2^- \rightarrow HO_2^-$ reaction, direct removal of hydroxyl radicals is a primary mode of H_2 action. There are no known enzymes that can specifically be used to treat •OH free radicals (Figure 1-4). Because •OH reacts almost immediately with cell biomolecules and is considered to be the main initiator of oxidative damage, the selective reaction of the H_2 gas and the ability to neutralize hydroxyl radicals are highly desirable properties.

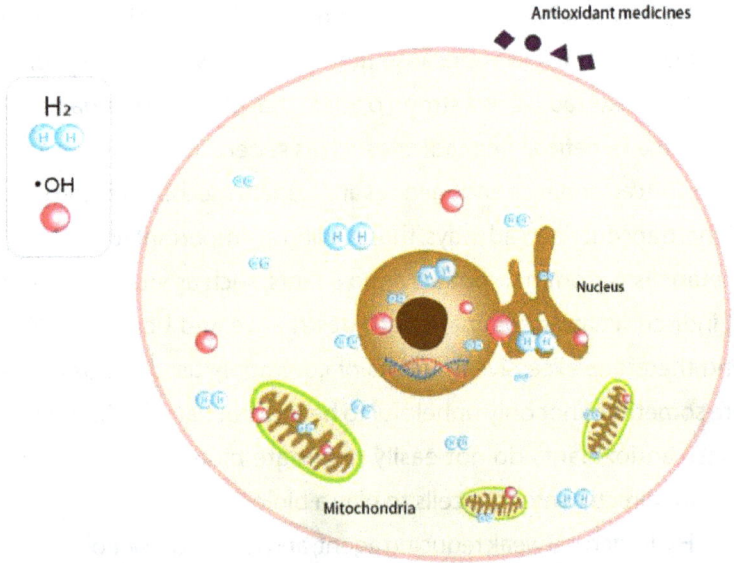

Figure 1-3 High diffusion of molecular hydrogen.

H_2 has a low molecular weight and can quickly diffuse through cell membranes and lipid bilayers, reaching the nucleus and mitochondria, while common anti-oxidant agents do not have this property.

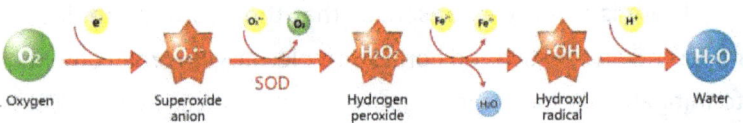

Figure 1-4 Production of ROS (•OH) by action of enzymes and effect of antioxidants and selective action of H_2 during respiration in mitochondria.

Many of the harmful consequences of the COVID-19 disease, including acute lung injury, can be attributed to hydroxyl free radicals. Therefore, the effect of hydrogen on scavenging the hydroxyl radicals can obviously alleviate various damages attributed to the hydroxyl radicals.

Further research found that H_2 exists only briefly in the body, yet it still maintains good biological and antioxidant effects even after being cleared from the body, This may indicate that H_2 may have mechanisms other than direct scavenging of free radicals.

The first, H_2 enhances the innate antioxidant mechanism. Catalase and SOD are very effective in detoxifying H_2O_2 and $O_2\bullet^-$, respectively, and can theoretically reduce ROS-induced cell damage. At the proper concentration, they can be converted into $\bullet$OH radicals through the Haber-Weiss and Fenton reaction in the presence of catalytically active metals (such as Fe_2^+ and Cu^+), preventing the generation of hydroxyl radicals. However, because these enzymes cannot cross the cell membrane barrier and are rapidly eliminated, they may have only limited clinical effects.

The second, H_2 modulates the nuclear factor erythroid 2 related factor 2 (Nrf2) pathway. An important mechanism of cellular anti-oxidative stress is the activation of Nrf2 antioxidative response element (ARE) signaling pathway to induce phase II enzymes. Nrf2 is considered to be an important regulator of electrophilic/antioxidant homeostasis, especially in maintaining functional integrity of cells under oxidative stress conditions. Imbalance of cellular redox status caused by elevated ROS levels and/or reduced antioxidant levels is an important signal to induce a transcription response mediated by Nrf2 (Figure 1-5).

Under stress-free conditions, Nrf2 levels in the cytoplasm are regulated by Kelch-like ECH-related protein 1 (Keap1 protein), preventing its release into the nucleus and preventing its degradation.

Under stress, the Nrf2 pathway is activated and can induce the dissociation of Nrf2 from the Keap1 protein, which transfer the Nrf2

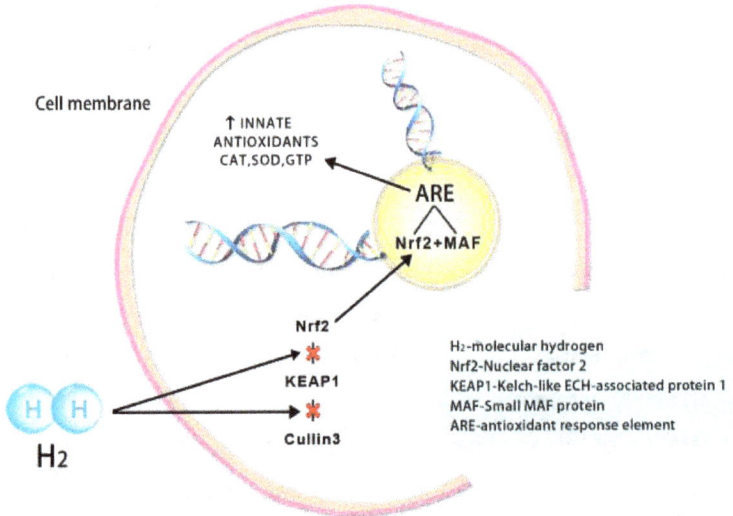

Figure 1-5 Mechanism of H_2 action: transcription and production of innate antioxidants upon entry into cell cytoplasm, release and accumulation of Nrf2 and its translocation into the nucleus.

CAT: catalase; SOD: superoxide dismutase; GTP; glutathione peroxidase.

From LeBaron, et al. [2019].

transcription factor into the nucleus, where it binds to the cognate DNA regulatory elements called ARE or electrophilic reactive elements (EpRE). Binding triggers transcription of antioxidant genes, leading to the production of many cytoprotective proteins.

H_2 can activate the Nrf2/EpRE signaling pathway, prevent lipid peroxidation, stimulate the production of the innate antioxidant SOD-2, and increase the phosphorylation of Akt kinase on Ser473, which is a cell survival signaling molecule involved in Nrf2 regulation. Many of the therapeutic effects of H_2 may be attributed to the activation of the Nrf2 pathway, including the role in reducing inflammation and suppressing apoptosis.

The third, another emerging vector for the biological effect of hydrogen is miRNA. Due to the imperfect pairing of the non-coding RNA with the target messenger RNA, the stability of the miRNA and/ or their translation efficiency can be regulated. They are believed to be novel regulators of oxidative and inflammatory stress, which regulate the expression of multiple redox-related genes. Studies have shown that abnormal ROS-induced miRNA levels can cause cancer by activating various oncogenes or silencing tumor suppressor genes. Radiation induces oxidative stress and affects the expression of several miRNAs, including miRNA-1 and miRNA-21. Up-regulation of miRNA-21 expression is associated with fibrosis. It is also associated with increased expression of protein kinase C, which is also associated with tissue remodeling. H_2 has been shown to attenuate radiation-induced abnormal miRNA expression in rats, including miRNA-1, miRNA-9, miRNA-15b, miRNA-21, and miRNA-199 [LeBaron, *et al.*, 2019].

Anti-inflammatory effect

Many cytological tests have shown that cells have resistance to applied attacks (such as toxins, radiation, damage, etc.) for a long time after H_2 disappearance from the culture system, indicating that H_2 has persistent anti-inflammatory effect.

H_2 may inhibit the infiltration of phagocytes into inflammatory sites and the subsequent release of reactive substances. The anti-inflammatory effect of H_2 is mainly achieved by down-regulating various pro-inflammatory and inflammatory cytokines, including interleukin (IL)-1β, IL-6, tumor necrosis factor (TNF)-α, and intracellular adhesion molecules (ICAM) -1, high mobility group box (HMGB) -1, nuclear factor (NF) -κB, and prostaglandin (PG) E2 [Nogueira, *et al.*, 2020; Nogueira, *et al.*, 2018]. It has recently been suggested that hydrogen can reduce inflammatory damage by down-regulating miR-9 and miR-21 and simultaneously up-regulating miR-199.

Current research suggests that macrophages play a key role in molecular hydrogen's anti-inflammation. H_2 may increase M2 macrophage-associated anti-inflammatory cytokine levels and reduce M1 macrophage-associated pro-inflammatory cytokine levels. M2 polarized macrophages are a key component of inflammation resolution. M2 macrophage polarization depends on cytokines. Activation of the IL-4/IL-13 signaling pathway can promote M2 macrophage polarization. H_2 may activate M2 macrophage polarization by stimulating the IL-4/IL-13 signaling pathway. Macrophage polarization is beneficial for tissue damage repair because M2 macrophages can both secrete anti-inflammatory molecules and produce growth factors that promote tissue repair and regeneration.

Yao *et al.* [2019] explored the renal protective effect of aerosol inhalation of hydrogen-rich solution (H_2) in a mouse model of sepsis. During septic acute kidney injury, renal fibrosis and renal tubular epithelial cell apoptosis are accompanied by macrophage infiltration and the production of M1 macrophage-related proinflammatory cytokines (Il-6 and TNF-α) in renal tissue. Aerosol inhalation of H_2 increases anti-inflammatory cytokine (Il-4 and Il-13) mRNA levels in kidney tissue, and promotes macrophage polarization to M2 type, thereby producing additional anti-inflammatory cytokines (Il-10 and TGF-β) (Figure 1-6).

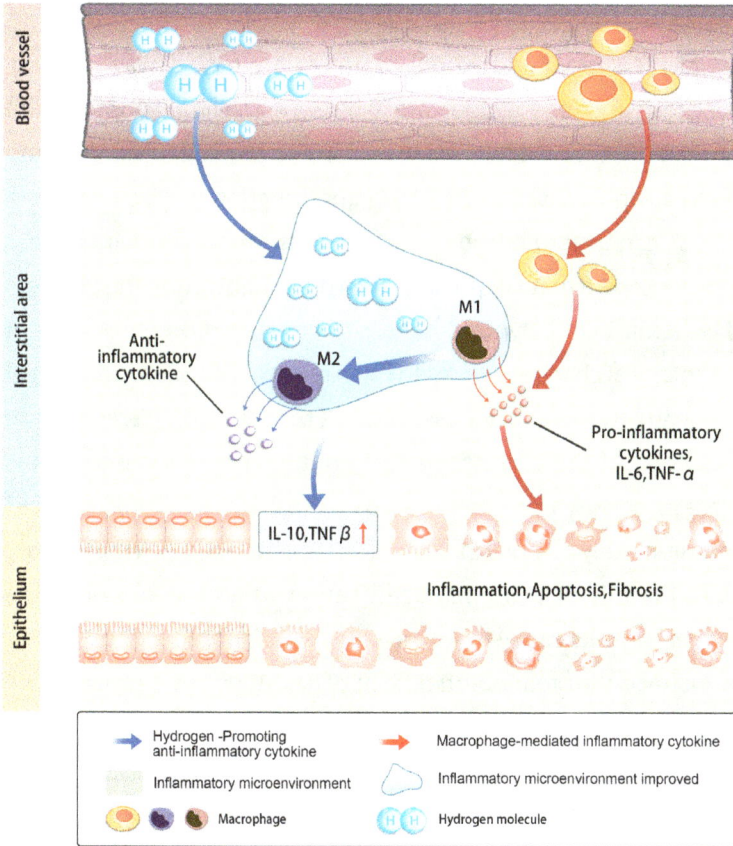

Figure 1-6 H_2 promotes M1/M2 polarization of macrophages and reduces inflammation of septic kidney injury.

Macrophages (Mf) play an immune function in the stroma of the kidneys. In the case of kidney damage, the permeability of vascular endothelial cells increases. Intravascular macrophages penetrate into the space, forming M1 macrophages that secrete inflammatory cytokines, thereby destroying renal tubular epithelial cells. H_2 can penetrate into tissues through blood vessels, change inflammatory factors secreted in the inflammatory environment, and promote the polarization of M1 to M2 macrophages. M2 macrophages secrete anti-inflammatory factors to repair damaged renal tubules.

Reproduced from Yao, et al. [2019].

Anti-apoptosis with cytoprotection

Apoptosis is programmed cell death, a slow, natural way of dying. Apoptosis and regeneration are in balance. Too little apoptosis, the number of cells can continue to increase to form neoplasm, but too much apoptosis, organ structure and function will be damaged, disease can be formed, and vital functions cannot be maintained.

It is known that apoptosis plays a prominent role in the progress of ischemic injury. Hypoxic-ischemic injury can promote a series of pathological changes in tissue, which result in ectopic expression of the death promoter Bcl-2-associated X protein (bax), leading to the formation of the apoptosome. Then, the apoptosome activates procaspase-9, which is followed by the activation of procaspase-3 and ultimately cell death. As members of the B-cell lymphoma-2 (Bcl-2) family of proteins, Bcl-2 serves as a class of apoptosis regulators at its early stages. Bcl-2 is an antiapoptotic protein that counteracts the proapoptotic effects of bax. Above all, an appropriate ratio of bax/Bcl-2 can maintain a homeostatic state in cells and ensure cell survival. H_2 could significantly suppress the expression of bax and caspase-3 and concurrently promote the expression of antiapoptotic protein Bcl-2, which strongly supports that H_2 has a cytoprotection activity [Zhu, et al., 2007].

Hydrogen can still activate the adenylate-activated protein kinase (AMPK) pathway, regulate cell growth, remodel energy metabolism, thus exerting an anti-apoptotic role.

There have been many in-depth discussions on the effects of hydrogen on apoptosis and cytoprotection in recent years. Three studies are introduced here.

Hydrogen and HO-1-Sirt 1 axis

It is known that heme oxygenase-1 (HO-1) has a cytoprotective effect through Sirtuin 1 (Sirt1) to form the functional module. HO-1-Sirt1 axis activation plays important roles in achieving H_2 cytoprotection. HO-1 is an important rate-limiting enzyme that promotes the degradation of heme and produces bilirubin and CO. CO has anti-apoptotic and anti-inflammatory properties and cytoprotective effects [Li, *et al.*, 2016]. Sirt1 is not only an NAD^+ dependent type III histone and protein deacetylase, but also a kind of long-lived gene that inhibits apoptosis and improves cell survival in mammalian cells. It is reported that Sirt1 reduces fibrosis in the liver and has a hepatoprotective effect. HO-1 induces Sirt1 expression by activating PGC-1α/ERRα. Sirt1 is capable of binding to the p53 which is one of the substrates of Sirt1, resulting in p53 deacetylation and lowering the ability of p53 to activate downstream genes, and ultimately reduces apoptosis [Nakamura, *et al.*, 2017; Li, *et al.*, 2018] (Figure 1-7).

Hydrogen and autophagy

Recent studies have also shown the cytoprotective effects of molecular hydrogen can be achieved by an increase in autophagy levels. Autophagy is an adaptive cellular response to "stress", in which longevity proteins, damaged organelles, and cytoplasmic content are eliminated to maintain homeostasis. Autophagy indirectly regulates intracellular oxidative stress by clearance of dysfunctional mitochondria and damaged proteins [He and Klionsky, 2009]. Autophagy dysfunction can lead to impaired mitochondrial function, accumulation of reactive oxygen species (ROS), and oxidative stress.

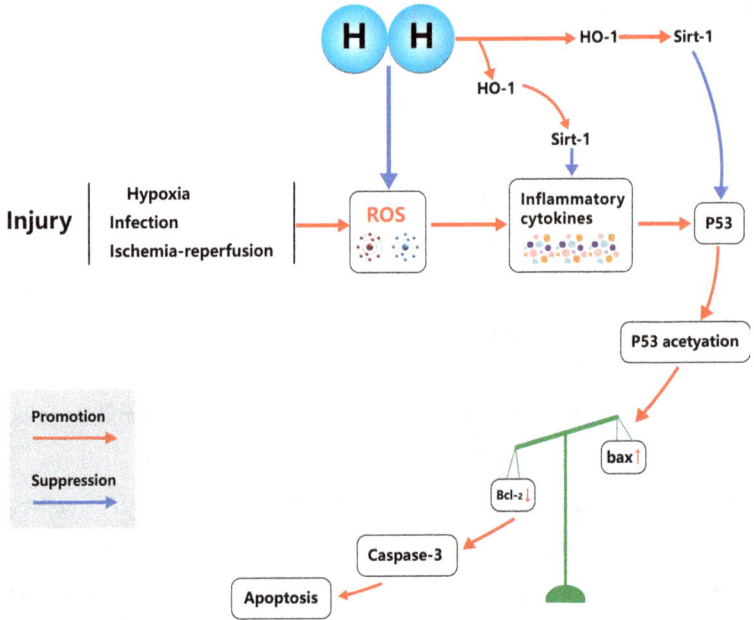

Figure 1-7 The schematic illustration of molecular hydrogen inhibiting apoptosis.

H_2 eliminates toxic ROS, down-regulating inflammatory cytokines. H_2 promotes HO-1 activity, increasing Sirt1 expression. Sirt1 inhibits the inflammatory cytokines and suppresses activity of the p53 pathway which directly decreases the Bcl-2/bax ratio and induces caspase-3 activation.

ROS consumes glutathione and causes protein folding errors in the endoplasmic reticulum (ER). When ER function is severely impaired, organelles trigger apoptosis signals.

Autophagy flux is inhibited in both ischemic and hypoxia injury. Accumulating evidence suggests that endoplasmic reticulum stress (ER stress) is activated in response to oxidative stress. ER stress is accompanied with the inhibited autophagy. The protective effects of hydrogen against ischemic/reperfusion injury is through inhibiting endoplasmic reticulum stress.

Beyond ER stress, mTOR may be involved in autophagy regulation. The mTOR inhibition increases autophagy. Activated mTOR may be responsible for lowered autophagy. Blocked autophagy is reversed by H_2, suggesting that the gas may play an important role in regulating mTOR signaling.

It is discovered that the p38 and JNK pathways are involved in the H_2 protective effects. Potential mechanism for the regulation of autophagy is via p38 MAPK signaling. The activated JNK can promote bax translocation from the cytoplasm into mitochondria, leading to cell apoptosis. H_2 inhibits the activation of p38 and JNK.

Taken together, apart from attenuated oxidative stress and apoptosis, H_2 mediates cytoprotective effects through inhibiting ER stress and increasing autophagy, which is at least partially dependent on the suppression of mTOR, p38, and JNK (Figure 1-8).

Hydrogen and blood vessels

Recent studies have found that the cytoprotective effects of H_2 also show its effects on blood vessels, including (Figure 1-9):

- In the angiogenesis pathway, hydrogen can inhibit the degradation of cyclic guanosine monophosphate (cGMP), by phosphodiesterase, leading to increased levels of cGMP, protein kinase activation, and angiogenesis.

- Hydrogen increases intracellular calcium levels and stimulates vascular endothelial growth factor, which in turn increases nitric oxide production.

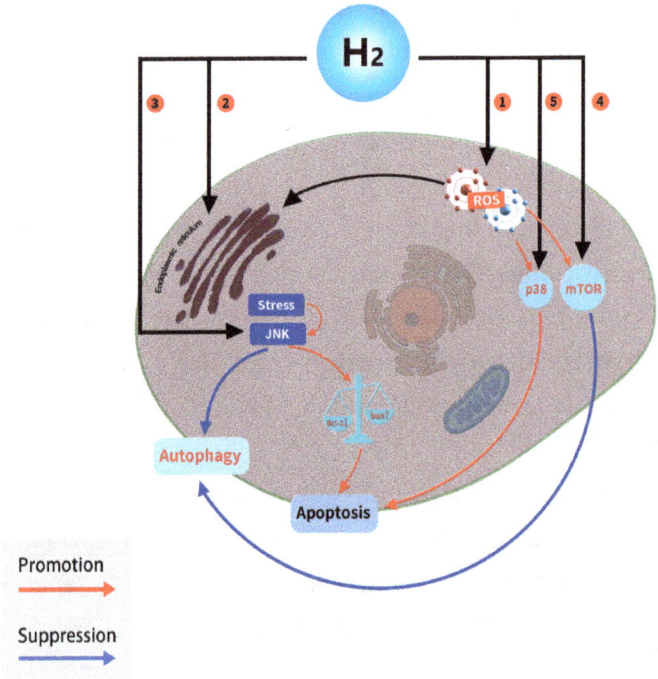

Figure 1-8 Proposed signaling pathways involved in H$_2$ inducing autophagy. ①Eliminates toxic ROS; ②Inhibits endoplasmic reticulum oxidative stress; ③ Inhibits JNK; ④ Inhibits mTOR; ⑤ Inhibits p38.

- Hydrogen opens potassium channels that are sensitive to adenosine triphosphate, thereby activating downstream mitogen-activated protein kinase pathways, including autophagy.

Hydrogen therapy with development potential may promote collateral formation of blood vessels through angiogenesis

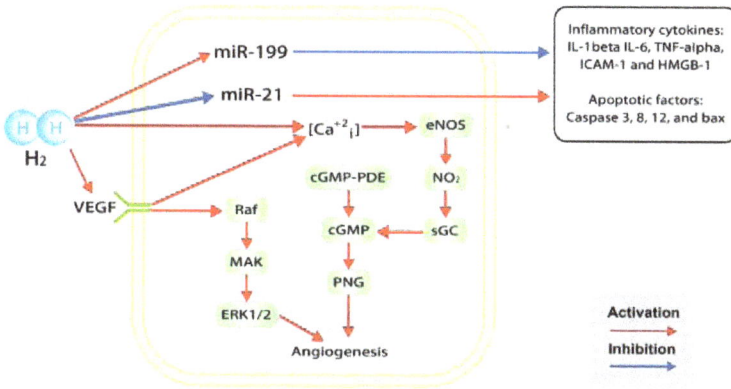

Figure 1-9 H_2 and angiogenesis. Proposed pathway for hydrogen (H_2) therapy and its downstream targets.

VEGF: vascular endothelial growth factor; MAK: serine/threonine-protein kinase; ERK1/2: extracellular signal-regulated kinase 1/2; cGMP: cyclic guanosine monophosphate; PDE: phosphodiesterases; PKG: protein kinase G; eNOS: endothelial nitric oxide synthase; NO_2: nitrogen dioxide; sGC: soluble guanylatecyclase; IL: interleukin; TNF: tumor necrosis factor; ICAM-1: intercellular cell adhesion molecule-1; HMGB-1: high-mobility group box protein 1. Reproduced from Zhu, et al. [2007].

mechanism and Flk1-Notch signal stimulated by paracrine VEGF. The increased collaterals in this microcirculation may be an important factor for H_2 to improve ischemic tissue damage.

Modulation of signal transduction

As already mentioned, molecular hydrogen exists only briefly in the body, and even after clearing H_2 from the body, it still maintains good biological and antioxidant effects. There is evidence that H_2 can regulate the expression of a variety of genes, including NF-κB, c-Jun N-terminal kinase (JNK), fibroblast growth factor 21 (FGF-21), and peroxisome proliferator activation receptor-gamma coactivator-1α (PGC-1α), proliferating cell nuclear antigen, vascular endothelial growth factor (VEGF), glial fibrillary acidic protein (GFAP), and many other transcription factors and regulatory proteins. However, these molecules are likely to be downstream or indirectly regulated by H_2, as the direct target of H_2 has yet to be elucidated.

As mentioned earlier, H_2 can regulate NF-κB. Downstream of this factor controls hundreds of genes related to cell growth, differentiation, development, inflammation, and apoptosis. H_2 can activate NF-κB, thereby activating a series of cellular behaviors.

H_2 can promote the expression of NF-E2-related factor 2 (Nrf2) *in vivo*, especially in organs such as lung, liver, and kidney. Nrf2 is a new regulator of the innate immune response. H_2 up-regulates Nrf2 and maintains the body's immune function.

As stated before, H_2 can induce heme oxygenase-1 (HO-1) and its enzymatic response. HO-1 and its product CO not only have significant anti-inflammatory properties, but also eliminate infection by increasing phagocytosis and endogenous antimicrobial response, and they can also reduce inflammation caused by hyperoxia and improve blood oxygenation.

Wang, *et al.* [2020] studied hypoxic-ischemic brain damage in newborn rats and found that the activation of HO-1 not only confers antioxidant effects, but also regulates redox homeostasis and regulates neuroinflammatory conditions in activated glial cells. PGC-1α has been shown to be essential in regulating mitochondrial oxidative stress and biogenesis. H_2 activates MAPK (ERK1/2, p38

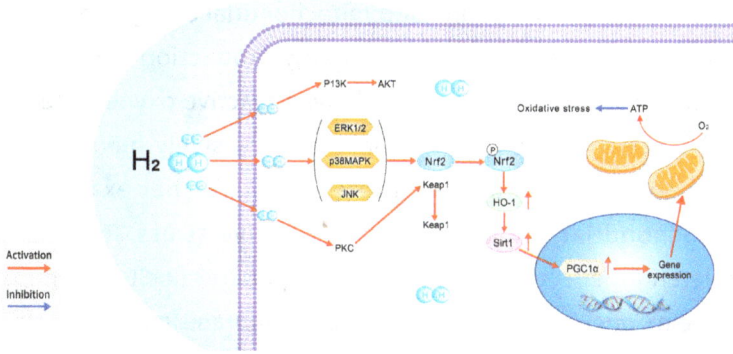

Figure 1-10   The proposed mechanism by which H₂ gas regulates the MAPK/Nrf2/HO-1 pathway.

H₂ gas upregulates the expression of MAPKs (ERK1/2, P38 MAPK, and JNK). HO-1 can be expressed by stimuli mainly via MAPK-dependent Nrf2 activation. HO-1 inhibits oxidative stress and increases Sirt1 expression. Sirt1 directly deacetylates PGC-1α.
From Wang, et al. [2020].

MAPK, and JNK) and increases HO-1 expression (Figure 1-10). H₂ exerts cytoprotective effects by regulating the MAPK/HO-1/PCG1-α pathway apart from reducing apoptosis.

Maintenance of mitochondrial function

Mitochondria are organelles with highly dynamic ultrastructure, which are maintained by flexible fusion and division rates controlled by guanosine triphosphatase (GTPases) -dependent proteins. The integrity of mitochondrial structure and function is essential for maintaining cellular energy and metabolic homeostasis. The dysfunction of fusion and fission kinetics can lead to loss of integrity and function, accompanied by accumulation of damaged mitochondria and mitochondrial deoxyribonucleic acid (mtDNA), which may stop energy production and induce oxidative stress. Mitochondrial-derived reactive oxygen species (ROS) can mediate redox signals, or excessively mediate the activation of inflammatory proteins, and further exacerbate mitochondrial degradation and oxidative stress. ROS has a deleterious effect on many cellular components (including lipids, proteins, nuclear and mtDNA, and cell membrane lipids), resulting in the net result of accumulation of damage-associated molecular patterns (DAMPs) that can activate pathogen recognition receptors (PRR) on the surface and in the cytoplasm of immune cells [Geto, *et al.*, 2020].

Mitochondria play a central role in inflammation. Under injury stress, the electron transport chain (ETC) becomes dysfunctional and elevated ROS generation occurs. ROS-induced damage may drive necrosis, leading to the release of cellular contents, including whole and fragmented mitochondria. ROS burst represents a major pro-inflammatory stimulus. The mitochondrial dysfunction and impairment of mitochondrial quality control processes may lead to the accumulation of intracellular oxidized components and their release as the cell DAMPs. The mitochondrial DNA (mtDNA), one of the DAMPs, is a powerful inducer of an inflammatory response, and has been proposed as a functional link between mitochondrial damage and systemic inflammation. These events bind and activate the following pathways (Figure 1-11) [Picca, *et al.*, 2017]:

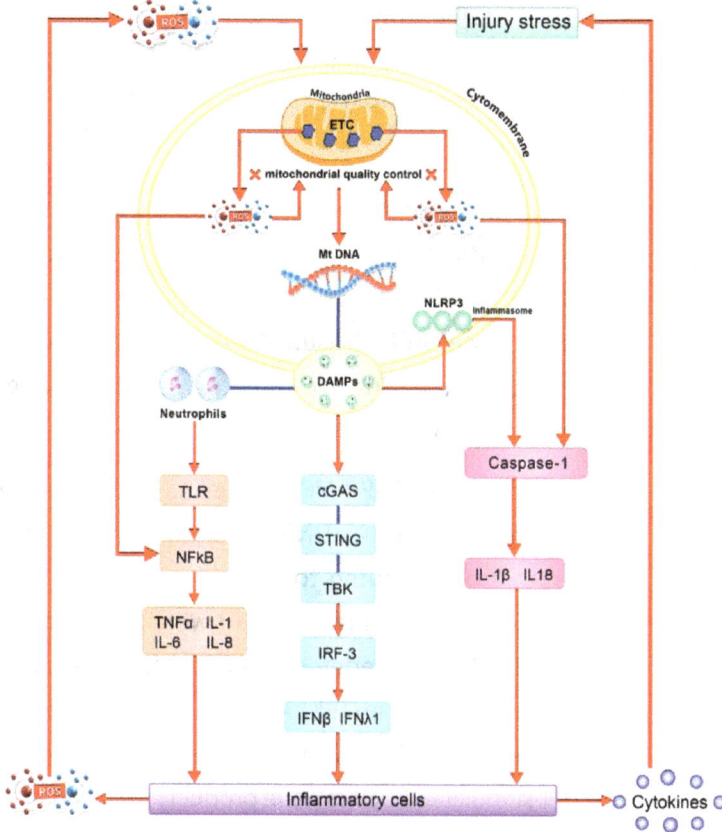

Figure 1-11   ROS, mitochondrial dysfunctions and inflammation.

The damage-associated molecular patterns (DAMPs) induce inflammation through activation of neutrophil-Toll-like receptor (TLR) and nuclear factor κB (NF-κB), the nucleotide-binding oligomerization domain (NOD)-like receptor (NLR), and the cytosolic cyclic GMP-AMP synthase (cGAS)-stimulator of interferon genes (STING) DNA sensing system-mediated pathways.

IFN: interferon; IL: interleukin; IRF-1: interferon regulatory factor 1; mtDNA: mitochondrial DNA; NF-kB: nuclear factor-kB; ROS: reactive oxygen species; TBK1: TANK-binding kinase 1; TNF-α: tumor necrosis factor-alpha.

(1) Toll-like receptor (TLR) and nuclear factor κB (NF-κB) pathway: the binding of DAMPs to neutrophils triggers the TLR followed by subsequent organization of the inflammatory response via NF-κB signaling;

(2) The nucleotide-binding oligomerization domain (NOD)-like receptor (NLR) pathway: DAMPs induce the activation of the NLR family pyrin domain containing 3 (NLRP3) inflammasome, which results in the engagement of caspase-1. The latter subsequently cleaves and activates interleukin (IL) 1β and 18;

(3) The cytosolic cyclic GMP-AMP synthase (cGAS)-stimulator of interferon genes (STING) DNA sensing system-mediated pathways: upon binding to mtDNA, cGAS proceeds through STING protein recruitment which triggers the transcription factor interferon regulatory factor 3 (IRF-3) via TANK-binding kinase (TBK). Activated IRF-3 induces the production of type I and III interferons (IFNs) (β and λ1) and IFN-stimulated nuclear gene products.

Inflammatory cells release cytokines, chemokines, and ROS in the circulation, and induce further mitochondrial damage, thereby establishing a vicious circle which reinforces the whole process.

By improving uncontrolled electron flow or preventing harmful electrons from leaking from the electron transport chain (ETC), mechanisms that can regenerate mitochondrial dysfunction are expected to regenerate cellular dysfunction by rescuing mitochondrial dysfunctional populations. Improvements in mitochondrial dysfunction are also expected to improve depending on cellular redox balance or disorder signals associated with it. H_2 can suppress the electron leakage in ETC, thus preventing the overproduction of superoxide, which is the first step in the process of mitochondrial oxidative stress.

It is suggested that H_2 activation and consumption in mammalian cells is mainly concentrated in mitochondrial complex I, which has a close evolutionary relationship with energy conversion membrane-bound [NiFe] hydrogenase (MBH). The possibility of H_2 serving as both an electron and a proton donor in the ubiquinone-binding chamber of complex I has been identified.

Ishibashi [2019] showed that when the accumulation of electrons leads to ROS generation, especially during the resupply of O_2 after mitochondrial hypoxia, H_2 converts the quinone intermediate to fully reduced ubiquinol, thereby increasing the antioxidant capacity of the quinone pool and preventing the production of ROS. H_2 has been proposed to act as a rectifier of mitochondrial electron flow in disordered or pathological states.

Ishihara, *et al.* [2019] studied the direction of electron flow, the production of superoxide, and the mitochondrial membrane potential, evaluating the role of H_2 in the mitochondrial energy conversion system (the source of reactive oxygen species). They discovered that H_2 only reduces the mitochondrial membrane potential of cultured cells by 11.3%. H_2 will change the direction of electron flow according to the ratio of $NAD^+/NADH$ and inhibit the generation of superoxide. H_2 can inhibit the superoxide production of complex I *in vitro* and reduce the membrane potential *in vivo*. H_2 can also neutralize semiquinone radicals to reduce superoxides produced in complex III. These studies suggest that H_2 can be used as a rectifier of electron flow that affects mitochondrial membrane potential to suppress oxidative damage to mitochondria.

Immunomodulatory effect

It is discovered that molecular hydrogen can restore depleted cytotoxic T cells and remove the body's immune suppression state, thereby maintaining immune balance in the body. Akagi and Baba [2019] reported that a total of 55 patients with stage IV colorectal carcinoma underwent hydrogen-oxygen inhalation 3 hours/day for 3 months. It was found that hydrogen gas decreased the abundance of exhausted terminal PD-1$^+$ CD8$^+$ T cells, increased that of active terminal PD-1$^-$ CD8$^+$ T cells, and improved progression-free survival (PFS) and overall survival (OS), suggesting that hydrogen can restore the balance between terminal PD1$^+$ and PD1$^-$ CD8$^+$ T cells by reducing the proportion of terminal PD-1$^+$ CD8$^+$ T cells. Xu, *et al.* [2020] gave 20 patients with advanced lung cancer inhalation of mixed gas composed of hydrogen-oxygen (67% H_2 and 33% O_2), 4 hours per day for 2 weeks, and found that almost all functional immunocytes, including Tc cell and Th cells as well as natural killer (NK) and γδT cells, increased after the mixed gas inhalation, while the multiple senescent or exhausted cell subsets decreased (Figure 1-12). Moreover, the proportion of Treg cells in the blood decreased.

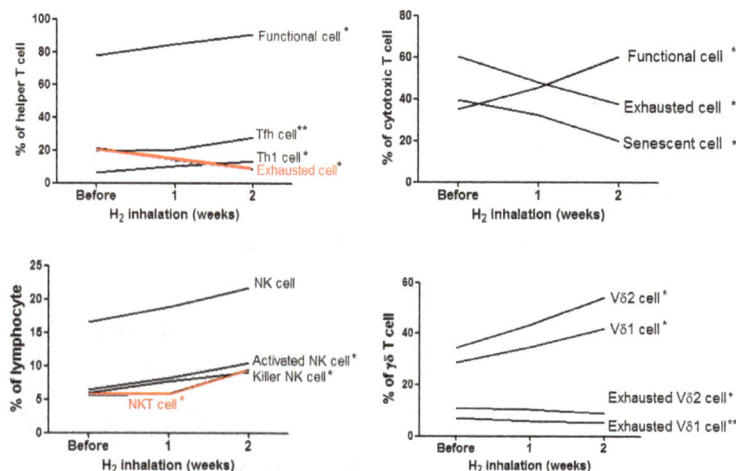

Figure 1-12 The change trend of immunologic cells before and after hydrogen (H_2 67% and O_2 33%) inhalation.

There is evidence that the regulatory effect of hydrogen on immunity may be mainly reflected in the rescue of exhausted T cells [Saeidi, *et al.*, 2018].

T cell exhaustion is a state of T cell dysfunction that arises during many virus infections and cancer [Wherry, *et al.*, 2007]. During acute infections, naive T cells are activated and differentiated into effector T cells. This differentiation is accompanied by the acquisition of cardinal features of effector T cells such as effector function, altered tissue homing, and dramatic numerical expansion. Following the peak of effector expansion and clearance of antigen, most activated T cells die, but a subset persists and changes into memory T cells, which maintain the ability to rapidly reactivate effector functions with antigen-independent self-renewal. If the infection continues to turn into a chronic infection, the programme of memory T cell differentiation is markedly altered, forming an altered differentiation state, termed T cell exhaustion, with progressive and hierarchical loss of effector functions, metabolic derangements, and a failure to transition to quiescence and acquire antigen-independent memory T cell homeostatic responsiveness. T cell exhaustion prevents optimal control of infections and induces overexpression in exhaustion of some inhibitory receptors such as programmed cell death protein 1 (PD-1) and cytotoxic T lymphocyte antigen 4 (CTLA4) (Figure 1-13).

In brief, exhausted T cells have the following features: (1) overexpress of several inhibitory receptors, including PD-1, (2) major changes in T cell receptor and cytokine signaling pathways, (3) display altered expression of genes involved in chemotaxis, adhesion, and migration, (4) expressea distinct set of transcription factors, and (5) profound metabolic and bioenergetic deficiencies. T cell exhaustion is progressive, and gene-expression profiling indicates that T cell exhaustion and anergy are distinct processes. It is suggested that functional exhaustion is probably due to both active suppression and passive defects in signaling and metabolism [Aubert, *et al.*, 2011; Crawford, *et al.*, 2014; Saeidi, *et al.*, 2018].

Reversing the state of exhaustion and reinvigorating optimal protective immune responses are of significant importance in clinical practice [Kamphorst, *et al.*, 2017; Saeidi, *et al.*, 2018]. It is known that mitochondria is critical in the regulation of innate and adaptive immunity. Immunity is required for T cell activation. Upon binding of the T cell receptor (TCR) with MHC, numerous signaling cascades are activated. An anabolic metabolic program is activated,

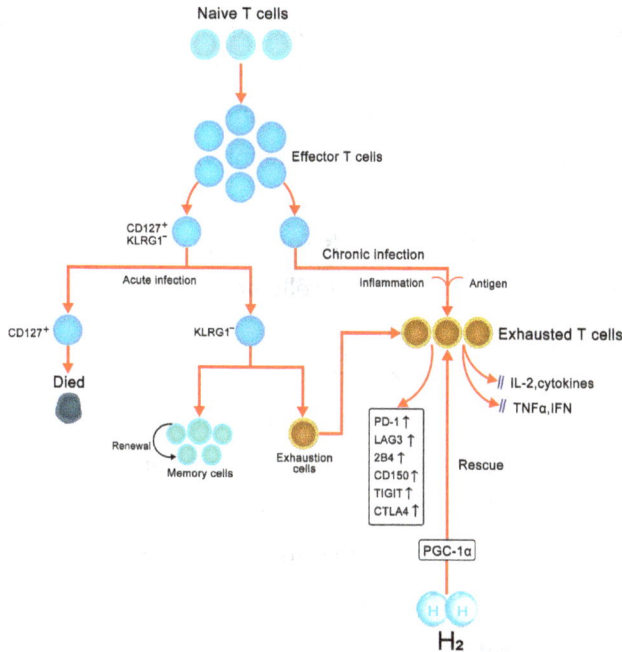

Figure 1-13   Development of T cell exhaustion after viral infection.

Upon infection, naive T cells are activated by antigen and inflammation, proliferate to form effector populations. Whereas the majority of effector CD8+ T cells that express killer cell lectin-like receptor subfamily G member 1 (KLRG1) die during the contraction phase, a population of effector CD8+ T cells that retains CD127 expression can turn to memory or exhausted CD8+ T cells. With clearance of antigen and/or inflammation, effector CD8+ T cells further differentiate into functional memory CD8+ T cells that can produce multiple cytokines, such as interferon-γ (IFNγ), tumor necrosis factor (TNF), and interleukin-2 (IL-2). During chronic infection, infection progresses and T cell stimulation continues, T cells lose effector functions in a hierarchical manner and become exhausted. Functions such as IL-2 production as well as high proliferative capacity are lost early, followed by defects in the production of IFNγ and TNF. T cell exhaustion is also accompanied by a progressive increase in the amount and diversity of inhibitory receptors that are expressed, including programmed cell death protein 1 (PD1), lymphocyte activation gene 3 protein (LAG3), 2B4, CD160, T cell immunoreceptor with immunoglobulin and ITIM domains (TIGIT), and cytotoxic T lymphocyte antigen 4 (CTLA4). Ultimately, if the severity or duration of the infection is high or prolonged, virus-specific T cells can be lost ("deletion"). Hydrogen (H_2) increases the gene expression of peroxisome proliferator-activated receptor γ coactivator 1α (PGC-1α), reversing the state of exhaustion and reinvigorating optimal protective immune responses.

Reference from Crawford, et al. [2014].

increasing uptake of glucose and glutamine to meet the increased metabolic demands of proliferation and induction of an adaptive immune response. The mitochondria in effector T cells functions as an anabolic hub where TCA cycle intermediates are shuttled into the cytoplasm to promote production of increase cellular biomass, while memory T cells utilize fatty acid catabolism to efficiently generate ATP to fuel cellular survival [Weinberg, *et al.* 2015; Scharping, *et al.*, 2016].

It is suggested that energy metabolism of mitochondria is depended upon the activity of a transcription coactivator called peroxisome proliferator-activated receptor γ coactivator 1α (PGC-1α), and FGF21 and PPARα, which are very important regulators of mitochondria. PGC-1α has a central role of activating various transcription factors in the regulation of cellular energy metabolism. When PGC-1α activates the transcription factor PPARα, fatty acid metabolism is enhanced. The PPARs function as ligand-activated transcriptional factors, all of which are subject to transcriptional coactivation by PGC-1α. PPARα regulates the expression of genes involved in fatty acid β-oxidation. FGF21 stimulates the phosphorylation of fibroblast growth factor receptor substrate 2 and extracellular signal-regulated protein kinases 1 and 2 (ERK1/2) to induce the hepatic expression of key regulators of gluconeogenesis, lipid metabolism, and ketogenesis [Weinberg, *et al.*, 2015]. The interactions among these key factors are complicated: FGF21 is PGC-1α dependently transcribed by PPARα, while FGF21 induces PGC-1α.

It is proved that molecular hydrogen increases the gene expression of PGC-1α as the early event. Thus, PGC-1α activates

PPARα, which transcribes the FGF21 gene and genes involved in fatty acid metabolism and steroid metabolism. In conclusion, PGC1α is a key node of signal integration, which links various cellular signals to mitochondrial biogenesis and T cell biology [Kamimura, *et al.*, 2016].

In addition, H_2 reduces hydroxyl radicals, which is a trigger of the free-radical chain reaction, so it should prevent the free-radical chain reaction, resulting in decreases of peroxides and their end products [Kamimura, *et al.*, 2016].

Also, CoQ10 may also be related to the immune regulation of hydrogen. Akagi and Baba [2019] found that 72% of patients receiving hydrogen therapy had elevated blood Co Q10 levels. CoQ10 is an indispensable electron carrier in the mitochondrial respiratory chain. It can transfer the electrons in complex I and complex II to complex III, catalyzing the combination of molecular hydrogen and •OH to form H_2O, neutralizing •OH, and reducing the damage of •OH to mitochondria [Xu and Chen, 2020].

It must be pointed out that the senescence of immune cells is concentrated on the phenotypic characteristics of individual lymphocytes, and the function does not necessarily decrease during aging. Unlike depletion, aging immune cells do not necessarily and gradually decline all immune functions, but are a highly dynamic process of remodeling and adaptation [Fulop, *et al.*, 2010; Akagi and Baba, 2019]. Hydrogen may play a regulatory role in this adaptation process.

Good and stable immune function plays an important role in clearing virus infection. COVID-19 infection is often severe in elderly patients and has a high mortality rate, which may be related to the exhaustion and dysfunction of immune cells. Hydrogen can rescue the functions of exhausted and senescent lymphocytes, which is obviously very beneficial in improving patients' condition and prognosis.

In conclusion, the above biological effects of H_2 are not independent of each other, but are interrelated. For example, H_2 can directly eliminate •OH, but this effect is related to multiple signal transduction. The reduction of inflammation is not only related to various signaling, but also due to the mechanism of altered gene expression. H_2 protection of mitochondria is related to apoptosis and immune regulation.

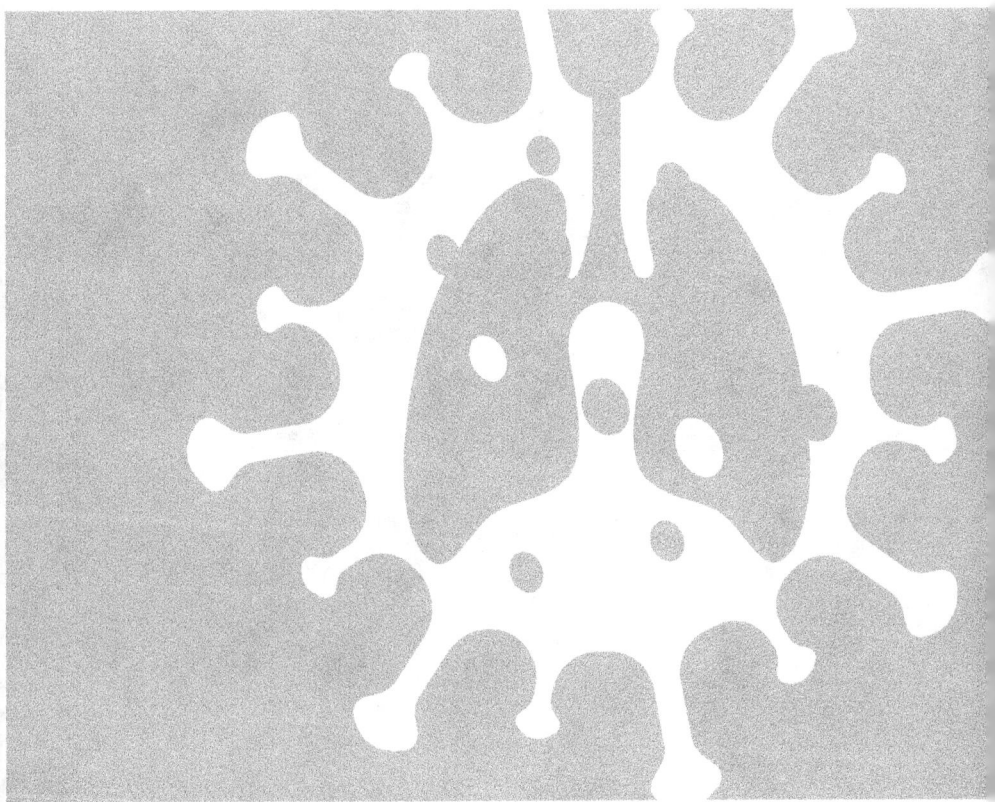

Effects of Hydrogen on Experimental Lung Damage

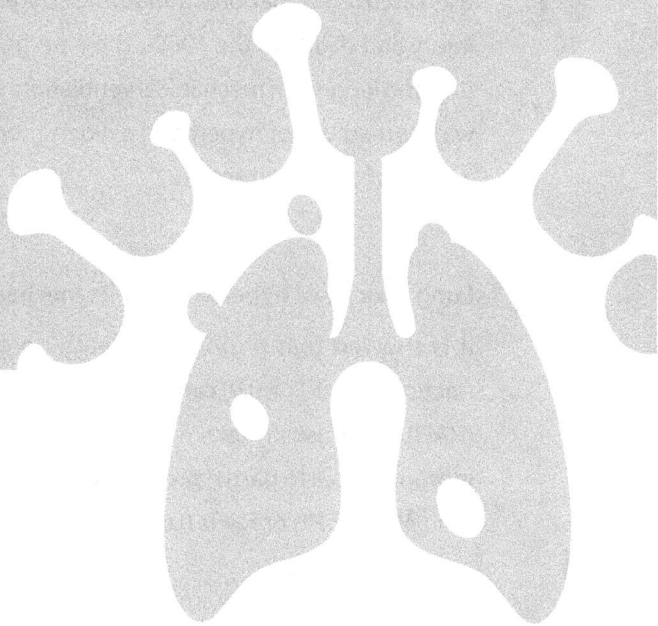

Acute lung injury (ALI) can be caused by a variety of factors, such as hyperoxia, mechanical ventilation, sepsis, multiple trauma, cardiopulmonary bypass, and viral pneumonia which causes acute respiratory failure and systemic inflammation presented by hypoxemia, lung infiltration, and edema. Oxidative stress, inflammation, and mitochondrial dysfunction play crucial roles in the pathogenesis of ALI [Fan, *et al.*, 2018; Chalmers, *et al.*, 2019].

Hyperoxic acute lung injury

In the late 18th century, oxygen (O_2) and its relationship with metabolism were discovered and quickly introduced into the treatment of cardiopulmonary diseases. Almost at the same time, it was discovered that breathing pure oxygen may cause irreparable injury and death. In the 1960s, the emergence of the intensive care unit and long-term mechanical ventilation, as well as the increasingly widespread use of hyperbaric oxygen therapy, made hyperoxemia a focus of clinical attention.

Lung toxicity of hyperoxia and its mechanism

It is showed that prolonged breathing of very high inspired O_2 fraction (F_{IO2}) ($F_{IO2} \geq 0.9$) can cause severe hyperoxic acute lung injury (HALI) and is usually fatal without reducing F_{IO2}. The severity of HALI is proportional to partial pressure of oxygen (PO_2) (especially higher than 450 mmHg or F_{IO2} is 0.6) and exposure time.

The earliest adult clinical report of apparent HALI was published in 1958 [Pratt, 1958]. Researchers soon correlated O_2 treatment with hyaline membrane formation in lungs of adults who died of progressive respiratory failure. Later, the formation of a transparent film was widely regarded as a hallmark of HALI. This was an important finding among patients who died of viral pneumonia during the 1918 influenza pandemic.

A meta analysis was done to determine whether any association existed between arterial hyperoxia and mortality in critically ill patient subsets. A total of 17 studies were identified in different patient categories and showed that hyperoxia was associated with increased mortality of patients with post-cardiac arrest, stroke, and traumatic brain injury [Damiani, *et al.*, 2014]. Animal studies showed that hyperoxia was associated with adverse events such as interstitial fibrosis, atelectasis, tracheobronchitis, alveolar protein leakage, and infiltration by neutrophils [Altemeier, *et al.*, 2007]. Human studies showed that hyperoxemia could weaken the responsive ability of the host's defense system to infections. In addition, hyperoxia could also lead to a decrease in cardiac output, coronary blood flow, and myocardial oxygen consumption [Tateda, *et al.*, 2003]. So far, many studies have shown that hyperoxia itself could trigger pathological conditions similar to ALI. Prolonged delivery of high concentrations of oxygen is suspected to exacerbate ALI in critically ill patients [Dias-Freitas, *et al.*, 2016].

The major advancement in the understanding of HALI only began in 1954, when it was discovered that abnormal ROS production was the cause of O_2 poisoning. The paradox of O_2 is that it is necessary for the life of aerobic cells yet destroys it by generating free radicals called ROS [Zhilyaer, *et al.*, 2003]. Hyperoxemia causes initial cell damage from the production of ROS through the law of mass action, where the production of ROS is proportional to the tissue PO_2.

Aerobic metabolism involves reducing oxygen molecules to form adenosine triphosphate and water. ROS is produced as an intermediate metabolite. In the initial stage of HALI, the most important source of ROS production is mitochondria (Figure 2-1). During oxidative phosphorylation, energy conversion occurs on three protein complexes. The inner membrane of mitochondria is called complex I, complex III and complex IV. Generally, 1–2% of O_2 molecules undergo "electron leakage" at complex I and complex III, thereby forming a small steady-state superoxide anion [Turrens, 2003; Janssen, *et al.*, 1993; Kallet, *et al.*, 2013].

The basic mechanisms for controlling the secondary pathway of ROS and hyperoxia leading to cell death include loss of plasma membrane integrity, the injury of mitochondrial membrane, releasing of cytochrome C into the cytoplasm, destruction of the nuclear membrane and DNA. Moreover, cell trauma triggers the production and release of pro-inflammatory cytokines and chemokines into the extracellular space and circulation, and attract and activate platelets, neutrophils, and macrophages, causing ROS explosion secondary to these inflammatory cells. Direct cell trauma leads to necrosis or "unplanned" cell death. In addition, the release of cytochrome C into the cytoplasm (A-1) and plasma membrane

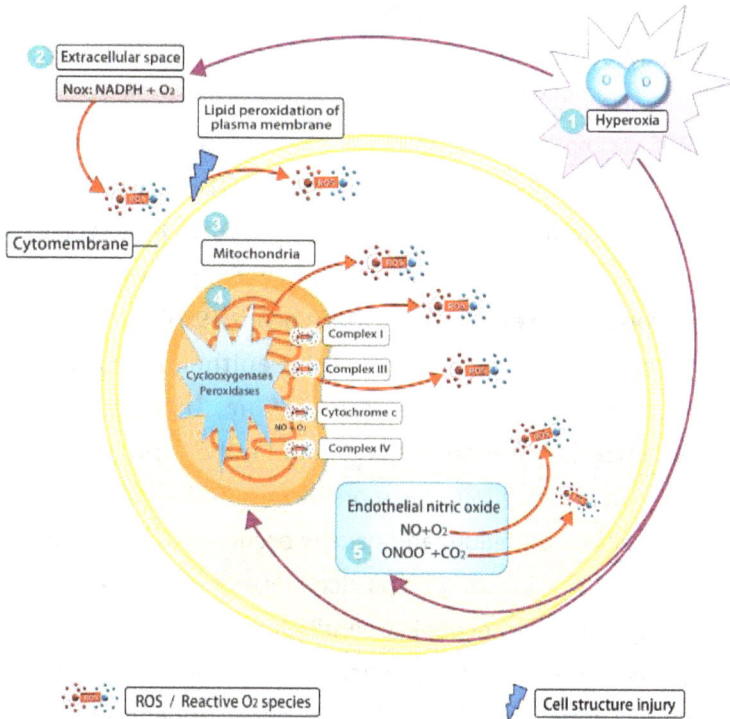

Figure 2-1 The mechanism of the initial burst of reactive oxygen species (ROS) induced by hyperoxia in pulmonary capillary endothelial cells.

(1)ROS generation is proportional to the partial pressure of oxygen (PO_2) during hyperoxia. (2)O_2 molecules are reduced to form ROS by nicotinamide adenine dinucleotide phosphate hydrogen (NADPH) oxidase (Nox) at the plasma membrane. (3)Damage to the plasma membrane lipid bilayer by ROS also generates additional ROS. (4)The primary sources of ROS production occur inside the mitochondria. Inadvertent electron leakage normally occurs at intermediate steps of energy transformation on the cytochrome chain (protein complexes I and III), but increases proportionally with the intensity of hyperoxia. Additional sources of ROS are generated from the interaction of O_2 molecules with numerous mitochondrial enzymes, including cyclooxygenases, peroxidases, lipoxygenase, and cytochrome P450. (5)The endothelium is a rich source of nitric oxide (NO), which react with O_2 molecules and superoxide anion to produce nitrogen dioxide (NO_2) and peroxynitrite anion ($ONOO-$), respectively. Peroxynitrite anion reacts with carbon dioxide to form additional NO_2.

Reference and reproduced from Kallet and Matthay [2013].

(A-2) damage triggers other cellular processes that instruct cells to essentially "suicide" (apoptosis) through the process of apoptosis [Pagano, *et al.*, 2003].

ROS has another important extracellular source, the nicotinamide adenine dinucleotide hydrogen phosphate (NADPH) oxidase (Nox) enzyme family, which uses NADPH to reduce O_2 to O_2 •-. Hyperoxia can increase the production of ROS through this pathway, which is proportional to the extracellular PO_2 [Brigham, 1986].

Hyperoxia damages the alveolar epithelium as well as macrophages and vascular endothelium. This response is characterized by enhanced alveolar capillary protein leak. Capillary endothelial injury is more extensive than the damage to the alveolar epithelium and usually occurs earlier. Pulmonary capillary endothelium may be particularly prone to hyperoxemia. In fact, high-stretch mechanical ventilation increases endothelial metabolism, which may theoretically exacerbate HALI, but that will be discussed later. The pulmonary capillary endothelium's susceptibility to HALI may be related to its high metabolic activity from regulating numerous vasoactive and fibrinolytic substances. This partially explains pulmonary dysregulation of circulating vasoactive substances during hyperoxia and subsequent pre-terminal hemodynamic instability.

Hyperoxia causes initial damage to the alveolar endothelium and epithelial cells, inducing them to release interleukin-1. This initiates the production and release of other cytokines, including interleukin 6 and interleukin 8. In turn, these cytokines stimulate the release of many other molecules that attract and/or activate neutrophils, macrophages, and other inflammatory cells, leading to increased vascular permeability and secondary ROS production.

The currently accepted view is that hyperoxia leads to excessive ROS production, stimulating oxidative stress and inflammatory response, which in turn leads to the destruction of alveolar epithelial cells, interstitial edema and type I cell damage, macrophage and neutrophil infiltration in the lung, and total lung volume decreases [Kress and Hall, 2014].

Another basic approach in HALI is to trigger apoptosis and necrosis. The former is through signaling molecules, the latter is due to trauma, such as lipid peroxidation of cell membranes, enzymatic dysfunction, and DNA breaks [Han, et al., 2018]. These two processes overlap through highly complex and redundant pathways, which ultimately leads to cell death. Apoptosis occurs both externally and internally. During HALI, the endogenous pathway is considered more important. Mitochondrial membrane damage caused by ROS and the release of cytochrome C into the cytoplasm are triggered, which in turn activates caspace-9.

It is discovered that apoptosis signal-regulating kinase 1 (ASK1), a member of the MAPK kinase (MAP3K) family, plays a pivotal role in hyperoxia-induced acute lung injury (HALI). ASK1 deletion *in vivo* significantly suppresses hyperoxia-induced elevation of inflammatory cytokines (such as IL-1β and TNF-α), cell apoptosis in the lung, and recruitment of immune cells [Fukumoto, et al., 2016]. ASK1 might be activated by oxidative stress through tumor necrosis factor receptor (TNFR).

Bhandari, *et al.* [2006] reported that the angiogenic growth factor angiopoietin 2 (Ang2) has an important role in hyperoxic acute lung injury (ALI). Hyperoxia induces and activates the extrinsic and mitochondrial cell death pathways and activates initiator and effector caspases through Ang2-dependent pathways *in vivo*. Ang2 increases inflammation and cell death during hyperoxia *in vivo* and stimulates epithelial necrosis in hyperoxia *in vitro*. Ang2 is thus a mediator of epithelial necrosis with an important role in hyperoxic ALI and pulmonary edema.

Moreover, hyperoxia also promotes alveolar epithelial-to-mesenchymal cell transition (EMT) through a mechanism that is dependent on activation of transforming growth factor-β1 (TGF-β1) signaling [Vyas-Read, *et al.*, 2014].

Experimental study of hydrogen for hyperoxic lung injury

Hydrogen, as a ROS scavenger, can relieve acute lung injury caused by hyperoxia. In order to determine whether hydrogen can reduce hyperoxic lung injury, scholars mainly from the USA reported a series of experimental results. As these studies involve the treatment of acute lung damage with hydrogen, which is discussed in this book, the experimental results of the researchers are described in more detail here.

Kawamura, *et al.* [2013] from the University of Pittsburgh Medical Center, USA, randomly assigned rats to four experimental groups, and showed that:

(1) *Hydrogen gas ameliorates lung dysfunction after hyperoxic exposure and prolongs survival against lethal hyperoxia in rats.* Sixty hours of exposure to a high concentration (>95%)

of oxygen impaired lung function, as was evident by the remarkable decrease in the partial pressure of oxygen in rats exposed to 98% oxygen. Administration of 2% hydrogen during hyperoxic exposure (hyperoxia/H_2) significantly improved blood oxygenation. All rats exposed to hyperoxia with 2% nitrogen died within 64 hours, whereas rats exposed to hyperoxia with 2% hydrogen survived a median of 72 hours.

(2) *Hydrogen reduces lung permeability, lung edema, and alveolar-capillary leakage induced by hyperoxia.* Exposure to hyperoxic conditions for 60 hours substantially increased the pleural effusion volume and the Wet/Dry (W/D) ratio of the rat lung tissue. Hydrogen ameliorated hyperoxia-induced lung edema, as indicated by reduced pleural effusion volume and by a significant decrease in the W/D ratio compared with lungs from hyperoxia/N_2 rats. The pleural effusion volume and W/D ratio findings provided consistent evidence that hydrogen reduced hyperoxia-induced lung edema. After 60 hours of exposure to hyperoxic conditions, the mRNAs for IL-1β, IL-6, TNF-α, and ICAM-1 were significantly upregulated compared with rats exposed to normoxic conditions. Treatment with 2% hydrogen during hyperoxic exposure significantly reduced the peak expression of the transcripts for these inflammatory mediators.

(3) *Hydrogen mitigates hyperoxia-induced lung epithelial cell apoptosis.* Prolonged hyperoxic exposure induced

apoptosis in the pulmonary epithelial cells. Hydrogen inhalation resulted in significant induction of Bcl-2 protein and upregulation of Bcl-2 mRNAs after 60 hours of hyperoxic exposure. The proapoptotic protein bax could be induced in alveolar epithelial cells by oxidative stress. Hydrogen inhalation reduced bax protein levels and inhibited the upregulation of bax mRNA.

Audi, *et al.* (2017) from Wisconsin, USA, demonstrated that inhalation of hydrogen can provide protection in rat models of acute lung injury using biomarker imaging. They used 99mTc-HMPAO and 99mTc-duramycin imaging showing oxidative stress and endothelial cell death, respectively, to track the effect of H_2 *in vivo* treatment. The results showed that lung uptake of the above biomarkers increased in a time-dependent manner in rats exposed to hyperoxia, whereas these increases were reduced to 120% and 70% in hyperoxic H_2 rats, respectively. Hyperoxic exposure increased the glutathione content in lung homogenates more than hyperoxic-H_2 mice. At 60 hours, the pleural effusion of hyperoxic-H_2 rats was also much less than that of hyperoxic rats.

Audi, *et al.* showed that lung histology from rats exposed to hyperoxia for 24 or 48 hours was indistinguishable from normoxia rats. Samples from lungs of rats exposed to hyperoxia for 60 hours exhibited variable degrees of edema, neutrophilic influx and, by high power, an increase in the width of the alveolar septum (diffusion barrier) relative to controls. Samples from rats exposed to hyperoxia + H_2 for 60 hours were not different from those of normoxia rats and were different from hyperoxia alone with respect to neutrophilic influx and barrier thickness. These data support that H_2 can provide protection against injury in rats exposed to only 60 hours of hyperoxia.

Hong, et al. [2016] found that in a zymosan-induced generalized inflammation model, the combination of H_2 and hyperoxic inhalation could increase the 14-day survival rate of mice to 100%. Moreover, the lung, liver, and kidney damage of mice inhaled by H_2 and O_2 was significantly less than that of the control group.

The principle of hydrogen improving the toxicity of hyperoxia

The mechanism by which hydrogen improves hyperoxic lung injury is thought to be its ability to selectively remove ROS. However, further research shows that hydrogen also triggers the activation or upregulation of other antioxidant enzymes or cytoprotective proteins to exert an indirect antioxidant effect, thereby protecting the lungs from hyperoxia. It mainly involves HO-1 and Nrf2.

It is known that HO-1 is a rate-limiting anti-inflammatory/antiapoptotic enzyme and catalyzes the conversion of heme into equimolar quantities of biliverdin. Free heme not only directly induces tissue injury of the lung cells but is also a major source of iron, which generates highly detrimental hydroxyl radicals through the Fenton reaction [Bysani, et al., 1990]. Hydrogen can induce HO-1 activity and increase the latter's conversion of free heme, thereby reducing lung damage.

Nrf2 is critical for the amelioration of hyperoxic lung injury by hydrogen. HO-1 induction by hydrogen is at least partially dependent on Nrf2. Moreover, the Nrf2-ARE pathway is activated by many different electrophilic and oxidative stresses and regulates a large battery of genes encoding proteins with antioxidant activities [Kensler, *et al.*, 2007]. Nrf2 signaling plays a critical protective role in pulmonary diseases such as carrageenin-induced acute lung injury. Nrf2 is also an important determinant of susceptibility to hyperoxic lung injury [Cho, *et al.*, 2002].

It was found that the transcriptional activation of Nrf2 is reduced under hyperoxic conditions, and if hydrogen is given at the same time, this decrease can be reversed. Hydrogen regulates the transcription of Nrf2 at least in part by regulating the Nrf2-ARE pathway, thereby exerting a protective effect on the lung.

Ventilator-induced lung injury

Acute respiratory distress syndrome (ARDS) is defined by the acute onset of hypoxemic respiratory failure. No effective pharmacological therapies exist for ARDS, and supportive care with mechanical ventilation (MV) remains the cornerstone of treatment [Fan, *et al.*, 2005]. However, MV itself can aggravate or cause lung damage, called ventilator-induced lung injury (VILI), which is one of major causes of mortality and morbidity of patients in the intensive care unit [Dos Santos and Slutsky, 2000; Tremblay and Slutsky, 2006].

In order to reduce such complications, the tidal volume is generally limited. But whether this measure can reduce VILI has not been determined so far.

VILI pathogenesis

The classic schema of VILI describes four central mechanisms: barotrauma, volutrauma, atelectrauma, and biotrauma.

The barotrauma caused by positive pressure ventilation has been recognized. However, most of the occurrence of VILI is not accompanied by clinically obvious barotrauma. Barotrauma and volumetric injury may be related aspects of the same phenomenon, and can be regarded as mechanical stress and strain, respectively. Atelectrauma refers to the injury caused by the periodic opening and closing of the small airways extending to alveolar ducts and alveoli during the period of tidal ventilation. In small airways, the periodic opening and closing of each breath will produce harmful stress/strain along the airway epithelium, because the opening of the airway is in an "unzippering-like" shape with air bolus propagation (Figure 2-2) [Madahar, et al., 2020].

Biotrauma refers to the biological response to mechanical damage. Regardless of the mechanism of VILI, mechanical cell damage will produce regional and systemic inflammatory responses, thereby promoting damage. Biotrauma is the final common pathway of VILI. After the bronchoalveolar epithelium and vascular endothelial cells are mechanically injured due to excessive stretching, a signaling cascade occurs. First, a damage-associated molecular pattern (DAMP) is released. DAMP is host-derived molecules that play a critical role in modulating the lung injury response within the airspace and interstitium [Tolle, et al., 2013]. The molecules induce the recruitment of immune cells, followed by the secretion of a large number of pro-inflammatory cytokines. Repeated exposure to harmful mechanical forces during tidal ventilation will further promote this

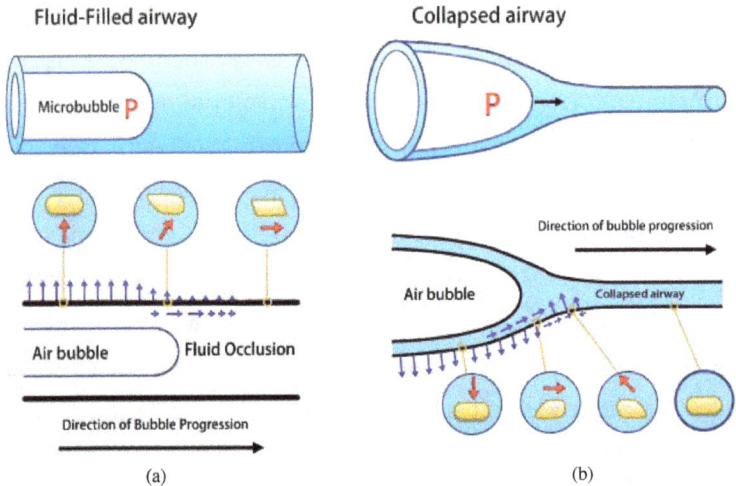

Figure 2-2 Schematic diagrams of local stress and strain of epithelial cells generated during recruitment of small airways.

(a) Air bubble propagation down the atelectatic airway generates a dynamic wave of stress and strain at the interface of the air bubble and collapsed airway. As the air bubble approaches, the epithelial cell is pulled inward toward the bubble. As the air bubble passes, the cell is pushed outward. (b) The air bubble similarly generates stress and strain of epithelial cells during propagation along flooded airway.

Reproduced from Ghadiali, et al. [2008]; Madahar, et al. [2020].

inflammatory process, thereby increasing the permeability of the alveolar capillary barrier, further reducing lung mechanics and predisposing to additional VILI in a positive feedback loop [Madahar, *et al.*, 2020].

Early in 1999, it was reported that patients with ARDS receiving mechanical ventilation had an increase in bronchoalveolar lavage concentrations of interleukin (IL) 1 beta, IL-6, and IL-1 receptor agonist and in both bronchoalveolar lavage and plasma concentrations of tumor necrosis factor (TNF) alpha, IL-6, and TNF-alpha receptors over 36 hours [Ranieri, *et al.*, 1999].

In recent years, the role of biochemical factors in VILI has been studied in more detail [Dolinay, *et al.*, 2012]. These mechanical forces induced by MV can activate macrophages and neutrophils in alveoli and interstitium and then trigger a complex array of inflammatory mediators, resulting in a local and systemic inflammatory response (biotrauma) which triggers detachment of endothelial cells from the basement membrane and synthesis of extracellular matrix components [Al-Jamal, *et al.*, 2001; Dreyfuss, *et al.*, 1998] and also promotes alveolar coagulopathy and fibrin deposition within the airways [Choi, *et al.*, 2006]. Inflammatory reaction propagates injury to non-pulmonary organs [Tremblay and Slutsky, 1998], which may result in multiple organ failure (MOF) (Figure 2-3). Research has shown that mechanical ventilation can lead to epithelial cell apoptosis in the kidney and small intestine, accompanied by biochemical evidence of organ dysfunction [Imai, *et al.*, 2003].

As MV can increase the level of inflammatory mediators within the lungs, treatment with inhibition of these mediators seems to be a reasonable strategy for the treatment of VILI. A number of potential targets have been identified in preclinical studies. Increased levels of several inflammatory mediators (including TNFα, IL-6, and IL-10) are found in *ex vivo* and *in vivo* VILI animal models [Frank, *et al.*, 2008]. It has been reported that IL-1 or IL-18 blockade mitigates inflammatory manifestations of VILI [Dolinay, *et al.*, 2012], and the prophylactic inhalation of anti-inflammatory cytokines, such as IL-10 and IL-22,

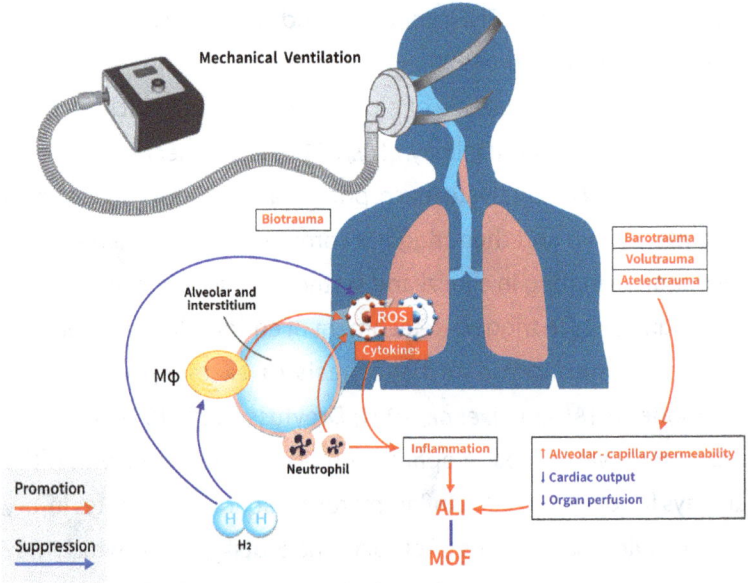

Figure 2-3 Mechanism of ventilation-induced acute lung injury and protective effect of molecular hydrogen.

MΦ: macrophages; ROS: reactive oxygen species; VILI: ventilator-induced lung injury; MOF: multiple organ failure.

Reproduced from Slutsky and Tremblay [1998].

may reduce or protect against VILI [Hoegl, *et al.*, 2009; 2011], but these have not been investigated in humans.

It is demonstrated that significantly increased level of the proinflammatory cytokine TNFα is in the alveoli following MV in a saline lung lavage of ARDS model [Imai, *et al.*, 1999; Takata, *et al.*, 1997]. Therefore, some studies examine whether pretreatment with intratracheal anti-TNFα antibody would reduce the magnitude of VILI. Following 4 hours of MV, levels of TNFα in the lung lavage fluid are significantly higher than at baseline. Pretreatment with anti-TNFα antibody reduces leukocyte infiltration, and ameliorates pathological findings in a dose-dependent fashion. However, given the complexity of the inflammatory response to MV and in ARDS, lung injury is not completely mitigated by pretreatment with anti-TNFα antibody alone. It is important to note that despite promising results using animal models of VILI, to date clinical trials of anti-cytokine therapy in critically ill patients have not led to any significant demonstrable benefit [Exley, *et al.*, 1990; Opal, *et al.*, 1997].

Obviously, a single anti-cytokine intervention for VILI will have no significant impact on patient outcomes.

Experimental study of hydrogen for VILI

Molecular hydrogen can theoretically improve VILI due to its antioxidant properties and broad-spectrum anti-cytokine effect. It is demonstrated that cyclic stretch associated with high-tidal-volume MV generates ROS and redox imbalance in lung epithelial and endothelial cells [Chapman, *et al.*, 2005]. The antioxidant properties of hydrogen to eliminate ROS may contribute to the mitigation of VILI.

Huang, *et al.* [2010] from the University of Pittsburgh Medical Center, USA, randomly assigned four experimental groups of mouse model. Mice under ventilation received the therapeutic (2% hydrogen) or control (2% nitrogen) gases via the tracheal tube. Results showed that:

(1) *Ventilation with 2% hydrogen in air exerts protective effects on the lungs and improves oxygenation of the arterial blood.* MV exacerbates inflammation and damage to the lungs,

which is clearly manifested by the thickening of the alveolar septum and inflammatory cell infiltration on histopathological examination. In the presence of hydrogen, both edema and inflammatory cell infiltration are reduced despite exposure to MV with a larger tidal volume and the lung injury score is significantly improved with hydrogen inhalation.

(2) *Hydrogen inhalation ameliorates upregulation of the mRNAs for TNFα, IL-1β, Egr-1, and CCL2 after 2 hours of MV.* This may explain the anti-inflammatory mechanisms afforded by hydrogen in VILI. Egr-1 acts as a key pro-inflammatory regulator in VILI. It is demonstrated that Egr-1-deficient mice do not sustain lung injury after ventilation, relative to wild-type mice [Hoetzel, *et al.*, 2008; Hilman, *et al.*, 2007]. The CC chemokine family is essential for the leukocyte recruitment during inflammation. Mounting evidence suggests that CCL2, a member of the CC chemokine family, is involved in numerous inflammation disorders of the lung, including VILI. Pro-inflammatory cytokines, such as TNFα and IL-1β, are elevated and play pivotal roles during the pathogenesis of VILI [Wilson, *et al.*, 2005].

Huang and his colleagues [2011] further demonstrated the molecular mechanisms by which hydrogen ameliorates VILI is related to nuclear factor-kappa B (NFκB) activation. The early activation of NFκB during hydrogen treatment is correlated with elevated levels of the antiapoptotic protein Bcl-2 and decreased levels of bax.

This shows once again that hydrogen plays a protective role against lungs during MV through anti-apoptosis and inhibition of inflammatory signaling pathways. This also suggests that it is reasonable to add hydrogen inhalation to the MV.

Septic acute lung injury

Septic shock is a common complication of infection, severe trauma, and major surgery. Immune cells in patients with septic shock are activated and produce large amounts of ROS which can increase the permeability of alveolar epithelial cells by destroying the cell membrane. At the same time, the accumulation of neutrophils in the lungs further causes ROS production. The lung is one of the most common target organs for sepsis [Fukuda, *et al.*, 2007].

As early as 2010, hydrogen has been reported to prevent and treat septic shock caused by a variety of bacteria [Xie, *et al.*, 2010]. Liu, *et al.* [2013] observed histological evidence of pulmonary hemorrhage, neutrophil infiltration, and overexpression of IL-6, IL-8, and TNF-α in septic shock in lung tissue, all of which are attenuated by hydrogen inhalation. Zhang, *et al.* [2016] also found that H_2 improves the endothelial permeability of sepsis mice by inhibiting the Rho/Rho associated coiled-coil forming protein kinase (Rho/ROCK) signaling pathway, and inhibits inflammation and oxidative stress, thereby reducing acute lung injury.

Dong, *et al.* [2018] explored the role of H_2 treatment in sepsis-induced acute lung injury (ALI) through various indicators. The results showed that 2% H_2 inhalation treatment can increase oxygenation index (PaO_2/FiO_2 ratio), increase mitochondrial-membrane potential (MMP) and adenosine triphosphate (ATP) levels, and up-regulate respiration control rate (RCR) and mitochondrial respiratory complex (I and II) activity and mitofusin-2 (MFN2) expression. It is suggested that H_2 improves septic lung injury by regulating mitochondrial function and dynamics. Liu, et al. [2015] found that H_2-NO combination therapy can more effectively inhibit the early and late activation of NFκB and lung cell apoptosis in lung damage, and significantly reduce lung damage induced by polybacteremia.

Li, et al. [2015], using the cecal ligation and puncture (CLP) septicemia model to induce severe sepsis, studied the effect of H_2 on severe sepsis and found that inhaling H_2 can improve survival and reduce the severity of lung injury by reducing the infiltration of inflammatory cells. Further studies have shown that the therapeutic effect of H_2 is related to increased expression of HO-1 and Nrf2, and the down-regulation of HMGB1.

Nrf2 may regulate an appropriate innate immune response, which determines the survival rate during sepsis. Nrf2 inhibits the inflammation reaction by adjusting the activity of its downstream protective molecule HO-1, which is a protective enzyme that plays an important role in inhibiting the inflammatory reaction [Gong, et al., 2013]. The increasing activity of HO-1 leads to the down-regulation of HMGB1. In the nucleus, HMGB1 plays a vital role in organizing DNA and regulating transcription. When sepsis damages organs or tissues, the mononuclear phagocyte system can release many types of pro-inflammatory cytokines and anti-inflammatory cytokines, including tumor necrosis factor a, interleukin 1, interleukin 6, interleukin 8, and macrophage migration inhibitory factor HMGB1. Among them, HMGB1 is one of the potential "late" proinflammatory cytokines in the pathogenesis of sepsis. HMGB1 expression is closely related to the severity of sepsis [Yang, *et al.*, 2014]. Mice with sepsis show up-regulated HMGB1 and inhibited Nrf2 and HO-1 activity in serum, lung, liver, and kidney. Angus, *et al.* [2007] find that HMGB1 expression is increased in almost all patients with community-acquired pneumonia.

According to above research by Li, *et al.* [2015], it can be determined that H_2 inhalation down-regulates HMGB1 by activating Nrf2 and HO-1 activity, thereby reducing the release of pro-inflammatory factors, thereby alleviating septic lung injury.

Recently, Yu, *et al.* [2019] conducted a similar study and also found that inhaling H_2 gas successfully reduces the morphological damage of lung tissue and the infiltration of inflammatory cells. They particularly emphasized that Nrf2 plays a major role in the protective effect of H_2 on lung injury caused by sepsis.

Chemical-induced lung injuries

There are many manifestations of acute lung injury caused by chemicals, including bronchopneumonia, pulmonary edema, and acute respiratory distress syndrome [Akira and Suganuma, 2014]. Hydrogen can improve these injuries.

Qiu, *et al.* [2011] reported that hydrogen inhalation can alleviate acute lung damage induced by lipopolysaccharide (LPS) in the trachea of mice, including improving the survival rate of mice, and reducing the lung wet/dry weight ratio. In addition, hydrogen decreases malonaldehyde and nitrotyrosine content, inhibits myeloperoxidase and maintains superoxide dismutase activity in lung tissues and is associated with a decrease in the expression of TNF-α, IL-1β, IL-6. Hydrogen further inhibits the activation of phosphorylate eJun N-terminal kinase (p-JNK), and also reverses the changes in bax, Bcl-xl and caspase-3. It is demonstrated that the protective role of hydrogen inhalation for LPS-induced acute lung injury may be exerted by preventing the activation of ROS-p-JNK-caspase-3 pathway. Ying, *et al*. [2017] applied it to oleic acid-induced acute lung injury in rats and found that hydrogen has a similar effect.

Liang, *et al*. [2012] demonstrated in the LPS-induced ALI experiment that hydrogen inhalation can reduce the expression of TNF-α in lung tissue and serum, and this effect may be related to the decrease of p38 mitogen-activated protein kinase (MAPK) expression and activation.

Xie, *et al*. [2012] found that LPS-challenged mice that exhibit significant lung injury is attenuated by H$_2$ treatment. Hydrogen gas treatment inhibits LPS-induced pulmonary early and late NF-κB activation. Moreover, H$_2$ treatment dramatically prevents the LPS-induced pulmonary cell apoptosis, as reflected by the decrease in TUNEL staining-positive cells and caspase 3 activity. Furthermore, H$_2$ treatment markedly attenuates LPS-induced lung neutrophil recruitment and inflammation, as evidenced by down-regulation of lung myeloperoxidase activity, total cells, and polymorphonuclear neutrophils in the bronchoalveolar lavage fluid (BALF), as well as pro-inflammatory cytokines (tumor necrosis factor α, IL-1β, IL-6, and high-mobility group box 1) and chemokines (keratinocyte-derived chemokine, macrophage inflammatory protein [MIP] 1α, MIP-2, and monocyte chemoattractant protein 1) in BALF. These results demonstrate that hydrogen ameliorates LPS-induced ALI through reducing lung inflammation and apoptosis, which may be associated with the decreased NF-κB activity.

Paraquat (PQ) intoxication causes lung oxidative stress damage. Zhang, et al. [2011] investigated the protective effects of hydrogen for acute lung injury caused by paraquat poisoning. Compared with the control group, the intoxication group had more serious hypoxemia, greater wet/dry weight ratio of lungs, higher malondialdehyde (MDA) level, higher expression of 8-hydroxydeoxyguanosine (8-OHdG), and more severe lung damage. However, after administration of hydrogen, poisoned animals turned out to have lighter hypoxemia, lower wet/dry weight ratio, decreased MDA level and expression of 8-OHdG, and milder lung damage.

Irradiation-induced lung damage

Terasaki, et al. [2011] investigated the possibility that hydrogen (H_2) could serve as a radioprotector in the lung. The acute and late-irradiation lung damage after hydrogen treatment was evaluated; the human lung epithelial cell line received 10 Gy irradiation and female mice received 15 Gy irradiation to the thorax. The results showed that H_2 reduces the amount of irradiation-induced ROS and levels of oxidative stress and apoptotic markers, and improves cell viability. At 5 months after irradiation, chest X-ray tomography,

Ashcroft score, and type III collagen deposition all indicate that H_2 treatment can reduce pulmonary fibrosis (late injury).

Lung injury after hemorrhagic shock and resuscitation

Hemorrhagic shock and resuscitation (HSR) is known to cause inflammatory reactions in the lung parenchyma and acute lung injury. Moon, *et al.* [2019] investigated the protective effect of inhaled hydrogen gas on post-HSR lung injury of rat model. Gas containing 2% hydrogen gas is inhaled only in the H_2/HSR group. The results showed that inflammatory cells infiltrate into the lung tissue more frequently in the HSR group. Myeloperoxidase (MPO) and pro-inflammatory mediators IL-1β, TNF-α, iNOS, intercellular cell adhesion molecule-1(ICAM-1), and CCL2, which are indicators of neutrophil infiltration, are significantly lower and there is minimal degree of lung injury in the H_2/HSR group than in the HSR group. Kohama, *et al.* [2015] did a similar study and found that hydrogen inhalation reduces lung injury after HS/R, significantly improves gas exchange, and reduces cell infiltration and bleeding.

Administration of hydrogen under hyperoxic conditions has been shown to be more effective in improving lung injury from hemorrhagic shock. Meng, *et al.* [2019] compared the effects of different treatment groups and found that PaO_2 and $PaCO_2$ in the hyperoxia plus hydrogen group have the most significant improvement, and the levels of serum lactic acid, MDA, TNF-α, and IL-6 have decreased. The morphological observation of light microscope and electron microscope showed that the cell damage is minimal in the high oxygen-hydrogen group.

Acute lung injury induced by seawater inhalation

Acute lung injury caused by seawater inhalation involves oxidative stress and apoptosis [Li, *et al.*, 2018]. Diao, *et al.* [2016] investigated the effect of hydrogen on acute lung injury caused by rabbit seawater drip, and confirmed that hydrogen inhalation can significantly improve pulmonary vascular endothelial permeability and reduce malondialdehyde (MDA) content and myeloperoxidase (MPO) activity in lung tissue. These changes are associated with a decrease in TNF-α, IL-1β, and IL-6 in bronchoalveolar lavage fluid (BALF). Hydrogen also reduces apoptosis, the expression of NF-E2-related factor (Nrf) 2 and heme oxygenase (HO)-1 are significantly activated, and the expression of caspase-3 is suppressed. They believe that the protective effect of hydrogen on the lung may be related to the activation of the Nrf2 pathway.

Lung injury after transplantation

Eliminating ischemia/reperfusion (I/R) injury is an important factor in long-term benefit for organ transplant recipients [Buchholz, *et al.*, 2008]. The Kawamura group [Kawamura, *et al.*, 2010] compared the consequences of inhaling different gases during surgery and one hour after reperfusion in mice undergoing orthotopic lung transplantation. Gas exchange is significantly impaired in animals exposed to 100% O_2, 2% N_2, or 2% H_2. Inhalation of hydrogen can alleviate the damage to the graft and significantly improve gas exchange. In the presence of hydrogen, the peroxidation of grafted lipids is significantly reduced, proving the antioxidant effect of hydrogen in transplanted lungs. Lung ischemia/reperfusion (I/R) injury results in the rapid production and release of multiple pro-inflammatory mediators and epithelial cell apoptosis. Exposure to H_2 can significantly down-regulate the production of pro-inflammatory mediators and induce anti-apoptotic molecules B-cell lymphoma-2 (Bcl-2) and B-cell lymphoma-extra large (Bcl-xl).

Zhang, *et al.* [2019] observed the effects of hydrogen inhalation on lung grafts during the warm ischemia phase in cardiac death donors. The results showed that exposure to 3% hydrogen significantly improves lung graft static compliance and oxygenation and remarkably decreases the inflammatory reactions and lipid peroxidation. Furthermore, hydrogen decreases apoptotic index and reduces NF-κB nuclear accumulation in the lung grafts.

Pulmonary fibrosis

Gao, *et al.* [2019] used a bleomycin (BLM) -induced pulmonary fibrosis rat model to investigate the effect of hydrogen (H_2) inhalation. BLM-stimulated rats show typical symptoms of pulmonary fibrosis, which is characterized by collagen deposition, alveolitis, and increased fibrosis in the lungs. H_2 inhalation treatment reduces the expression of transforming growth factor β-1 (TGF-β1) and TNF-α, increases the expression of epithelial cell marker E-cadherin, and down-regulates the expression of mesenchymal cell marker vimentin, suggesting that the epithelial-mesenchymal transition process is reversed. H_2 also down-regulates the expression of α-smooth muscle actin (α-SMA) and inhibits the production of collagen I, exerting an anti-fibrotic effect. It is proved that hydrogen inhalation therapy attenuates pulmonary fibrosis by inhibiting TGFβ-1, relevant oxidative stress, and epithelial-to-mesenchymal transition.

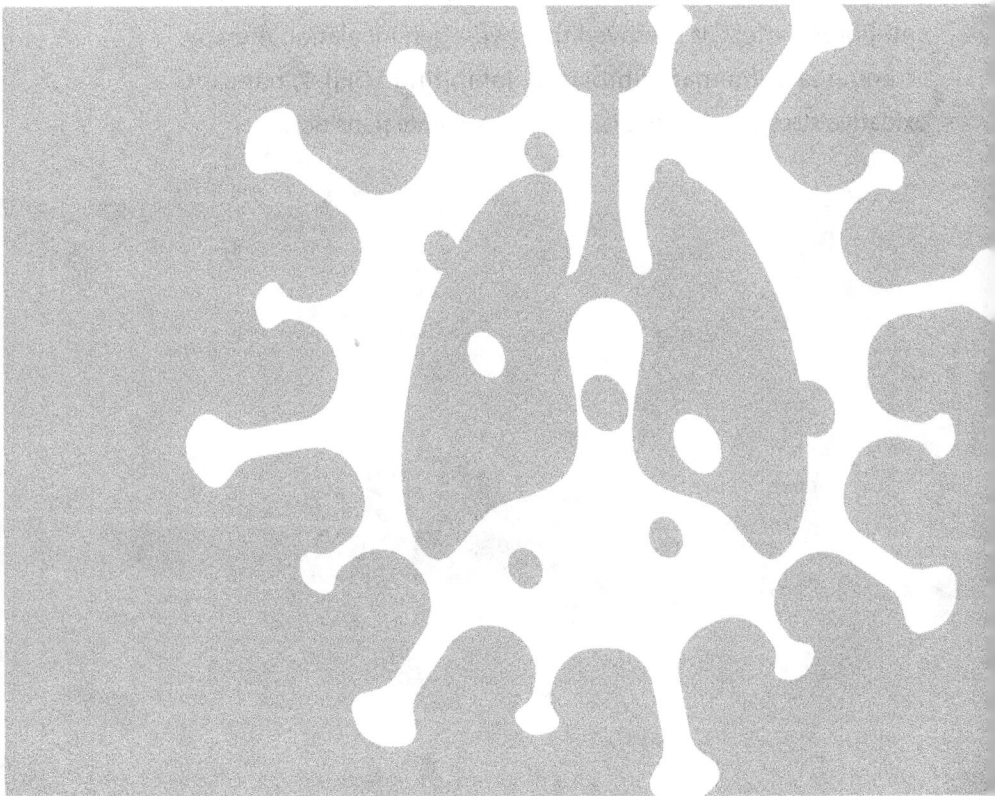

Pathogenesis of Viral Infectious Lung Diseases

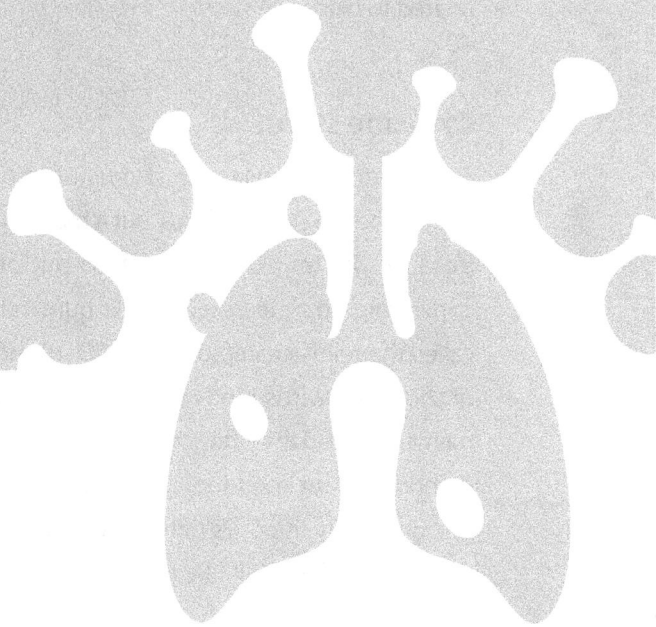

Among human coronaviruses (HCoVs), the severe acute respiratory syndrome coronavirus (SARS-CoV) and the Middle East respiratory syndrome coronavirus (MERS-CoV) together with COVID-19 pose huge threats to global public health [Liu, *et al.*, 2020]. They are polycistronic positive-strand RNA viruses, containing a genome of about 30 kb, encoding a variety of non-structural proteins (ORF1a and ORF1b) and a number of specific auxiliary proteins (such as ORF3a, ORF3b, ORF6, ORF7a, ORF7b ORF8a, ORF8b, and ORF9b) [Kannan, *et al.*, 2020]. The genomic sequences of the three coronaviruses are highly identical and highly pathogenic. In the pathogenesis, especially in the case of acute respiratory failure, the following mechanisms work: cytokine storm, apoptosis and necrosis, immunopathology, and fibrosis. The activation of all four might be related to oxidative stress.

Cytokine storm

The immune response against virus infection is the main mechanism for the body to clear the virus, but it may also lead to immune disease because the immune response is out of control. Angiotensin I converting enzyme (ACE2) in the human lower respiratory tract is called the cellular receptor for COVID-19 and SARS-CoV. The S protein of the coronavirus binds to the host cell via ACE2, fuses with the membrane, and the viral genomic RNA is released into the cytoplasm. Pathogen-associated molecular patterns (PAMPs) of viral RNA are recognized by the cell's pattern recognition receptors (PRR). These receptors include Toll-like receptors (TLR) 3, TLR7, TLR8, and TLR9, which sense viral RNA and DNA in endosomes. Viral RNA receptor retinoic-acid inducible gene I (RIG-1), cytosolic receptor melanoma differentiation-associated gene 5 (MDA5), and nucleotidyltransferase cyclic GMP-AMP synthase (cGAS) recognize viral RNA and DNA in the cytoplasm. A group of complex signaling recruit adaptors, including TIR-domain-containing adaptor proteins, such as IFN-β, mitochondrial antiviral-signalling protein (MAVS), and the stimulator of interferon genes protein (STING), can trigger downstream cascade molecules (adaptor molecule MyD88), leading to the activation of transcription factor NF-κB and interferon regulatory factor 3 (IRF3), as well as up-regulation of type I interferon (IFN-α/β) and a series of pro-inflammatory cytokines. If the above processes cannot be precisely regulated, or the host's innate immunity is abnormal, immune lesions will occur [Guo, *et al.*, 2020; Fung, *et al.*, 2020; Wong, *et al.*, 2004].

He, *et al.* [2006] detected MCP-1, TGF-β1, TNF-α, IL-1 β, and IL-6 in autopsy tissues of patients who died of SARS. High levels of pro-inflammatory cytokines are expressed in SARS-CoV infected ACE2-positive lung cells and cells of other organs, but not in uninfected cells, suggesting that a large number of pro-inflammatory factors produced by SARS-CoV infected cells induce immune-mediated damage, which not only lead to acute lung injury, but also multiple organ failure.

Wong, *et al.* [2004] investigated changes in plasma T helper (Th) cell cytokines, inflammatory cytokines, and chemokines in patients with SARS. Cytokine profile of SARS patients showed marked elevation of Th1 cytokine interferon (IFN)-gamma, inflammatory cytokines interleukin (IL)-1, IL-6, and IL-12 for at least 2 weeks after disease onset. The chemokine profile demonstrates significant elevation of neutrophil chemokine IL-8, monocyte chemoattractant protein-1 (MCP-1), and Th1 chemokine IFN-gamma-inducible protein-10 (IP-10). Together, the elevation of Th1 cytokine IFN-gamma, inflammatory cytokines IL-1, IL-6, and IL-12, and chemokines IL-8, MCP-1, and IP-10, all confirm the activation of Th1 cell-mediated immunity and hyperinnate inflammatory response in SARS through the accumulation of monocytes/macrophages and neutrophils.

Huang, *et al*. [2020] observed elevated plasma cytokines and chemokines in patients with COVID-19, including IL-1, IL-2, IL-4, IL-7, IL-10, IL-12, IL-13, IL-17, granulocyte colony stimulating factor (GCSF), macrophage colony-stimulating factor (MCSF), IP-10, MCP-1, MIP-1α, hepatocyte growth factor (HGF), IFN-γ, and TNF-α, which are shown as "cytokine storm". The anatomy report of COVID-19 pneumonia cadaver showed that the patient's lesions are mainly manifested by lower respiratory inflammatory response and lung injury. It is reasonable to speculate that after entering the respiratory tract, the virus particles mainly infect the lower respiratory tract cells, triggering a series of immune responses. If this immune process is out of control, a cytokine storm in the body will occur, leading to the seriousness of the disease

Xiong, *et al*. [2020] carried out transcriptome sequencing of the RNAs isolated from the bronchoalveolar lavage fluid (BALF) and peripheral blood mononuclear cells (PBMC) specimens of COVID-19 patients. The results show distinct host inflammatory cytokine profiles of SARS-CoV-2 infection in patients, and highlight the association between COVID-19 pathogenesis and excessive cytokine release such as CCL2/MCP-1, CXCL10/IP-10, CCL3/MIP-1A, and CCL4/MIP1B.

The proposed mechanism of cytokine storm caused by COVID-19 infection is summarized in Figure 3-1 below. In this process, ROS plays an initial and critical role. The ROS and its mediated oxidative stress will be discussed in detail in Chapter 4.

Apoptosis, necrosis, and autophagy

In addition to the cytokine storms observed in highly pathogenic HCoV infection, other cell death programs (such as apoptosis and necrosis) may also promote morbidity. Autopsy studies of SARS casualties have shown that a large number of organs, including liver and thyroid, have undergone massive apoptosis [Krähling, *et al.*, 2009]. Apoptosis induced by infection of SARS-CoV, MERS-CoV, or other HCoVs is described in various *in vitro* systems and animal models [Fung and Liu, 2019]. Apart from respiratory epithelial cells, HCoVs also infect and induce apoptosis in a variety of other cell types. For example, HCoV-OC43 induces apoptosis in neuronal cells [Favreau, *et al.*, 2012], while MERS-CoV induces apoptosis in primary T lymphocytes [Chu, *et al.*, 2016]. HCoV-229E infection also causes massive cell death in dendritic cells, albeit independent of apoptosis induction. The induction of cell death in these immune cells explains the lymphopenia observed in some HCoV diseases (such as SARS) and may contribute to the suppression of host immune response.

The mechanism of apoptosis caused by HCoV infection may vary according to the kind of virus (Figure 3-2). SARS coronavirus is

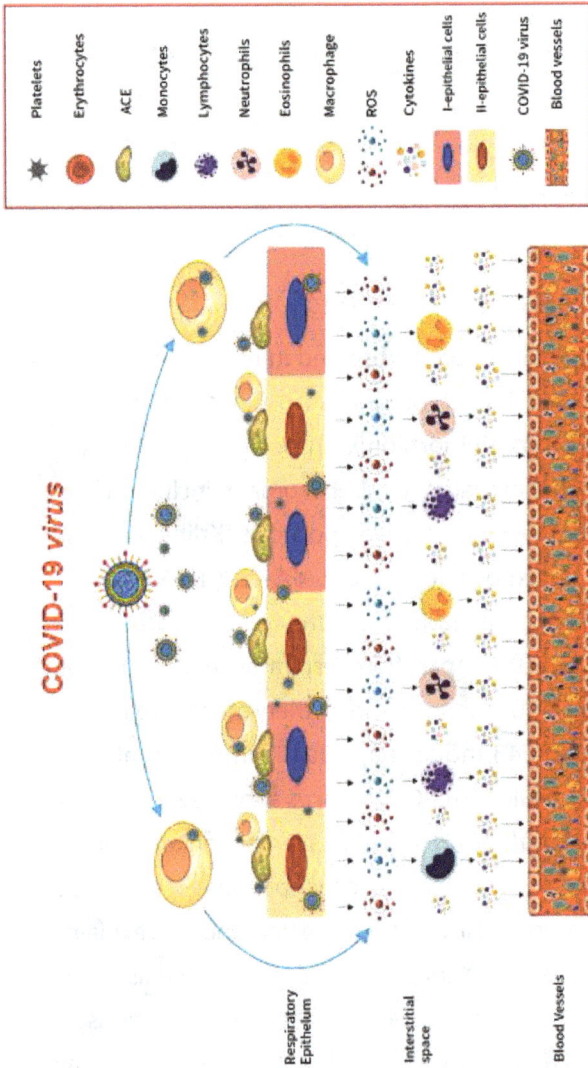

Figure 3-1 Proposed model of cytokine storm in COVID-19.

COVID-19 first enters inflammatory macrophages in the lung, which releases reactive oxygen species (ROS). At the same time, COVID-19 can directly enter lung epithelial cells through pulmonary ACE, destroy mitochondria and ribosomes in the epithelial cells, which produce ROS. Oxidative stress mediated by ROS mainly stimulates various inflammatory cells in the interstitial space of the lung to release a large number of various types of cytokines, causing a so-called cytokine storm or inflammatory storm. Interstitial ROS and cytokines can enter the bloodstream and affect various organs throughout the body. ROS, cytokines, and inflammatory cells promote each other to form a vicious cycle

ACE: Angiotensin I converting enzyme.

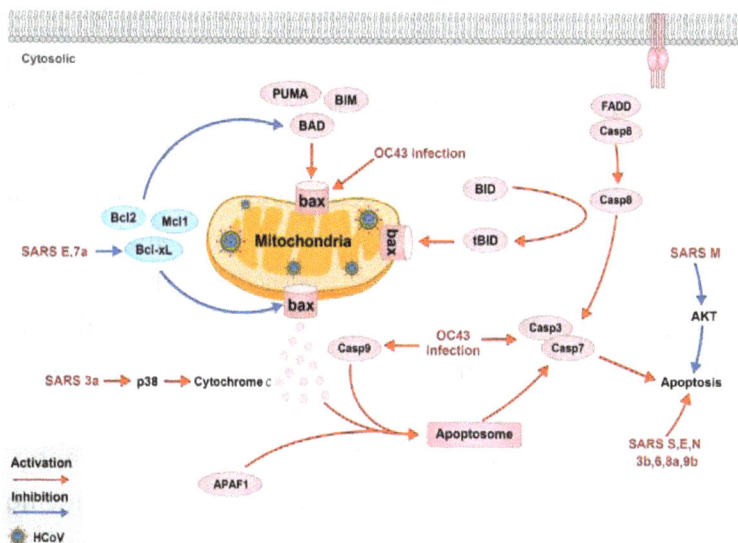

Figure 3-2 Apoptosis induced by HCoV infection and modulatory mechanisms.

Schematic diagram showing the signaling pathway of intrinsic and extrinsic apoptosis induction and the modulatory mechanisms utilized by HCoV.

AKT: RAC-alpha serine/threonine protein kinase; APAF1: apoptotic peptidase-activating factor 1; BAD: Bcl2-associated agonist of cell death; bax: Bcl2-associated X; Bcl-xl: Bcl-2-like protein 1; Bcl2: B cell lymphoma 2; BID: BH3-interacting domain death agonist; BIM: Bcl2-interacting mediator of cell death; Casp: caspase; FADD: fas associated via death domain; FasL: fas ligand; HCoV: human coronavirus; Mcl1: myeloid cell leukemia 1; PUMA: p53-upregulated modulator of apoptosis; SARS: severe acute respiratory syndrome; TNF-α: tumor necrosis factor alpha. Reproduced from Fung and Liu [2019].

originally shown to induce caspase-dependent apoptosis, which is virus-dependent but do not required replication. Although MERS-CoV infection of human primary T lymphocytes is abortive, apoptosis is induced via activation of both intrinsic and extrinsic pathways. Apoptosis of neurons infected with HCoV-OC43 is associated with mitochondrial translocation of bax, and is not related to caspase activation. In cells overexpressing SARS-CoV proteins, including S, E, M, N, and accessory protein 3a, 3b, 6, 7a, 8a, and 9b, apoptosis is also induced [Liu, *et al.*, 2014]. Among them, SARS-CoV E and 7a proteins activate the intrinsic pathway by chelating anti-apoptotic Bcl-Xl to endoplasmic reticulum (ER). Other pro-apoptotic mechanisms of SARS-CoV include interference with the survival signal of M protein and ion channel activity of E and 3a [Liu, *et al.*, 2014]. HCoV infection also induces apoptosis by activating the endoplasmic reticulum stress response and the mitogen-activated protein kinase (MAPK) pathway [Fung and Liu, 2019].

In addition to apoptosis, SARS-CoV also induces receptor-interacting protein 3 (RIP3)-mediated necrosis by inducing oligomerization of ORF3a. The higher the virus's pathogenicity, the more effectively it can activate different cell death programs [Fung, *et al.*, 2020].

As mentioned above, autophagy means that intracellular components (such as protein aggregates and damaged organelles) are engulfed into a double-membrane structure called autophagosomes, and finally fused with lysosomes to form autolysosomes for degradation [Yang, *et al.*, 2020]. It is suggested that activation by ROS and inflammasome is negatively regulated by autophagy/mitophagy [Nakahira, *et al.*, 2011; Saitoh, *et al.*, 2008]. Autophagy/mitophagy indirectly regulates intracellular oxidative stress by clearance of dysfunctional mitochondria and damaged proteins [He, *et al.*, 2009]. Macrophages isolated from mice deficient in the autophagy proteins have enhanced inflammasome activation and produce higher IL-1β and IL-18 [Nakahira, *et al.*, 2011; Saitoh, *et al.*, 2008].

There is evidence suggesting the possible inhibitory effect of HCoV on the autophagy process.

SARS-CoV contains the membrane-associated papain-like protease PLP2 (PLP2-TM) which is a nonstructural protein. PLP2-TM may increase the accumulation of autophagosomes but block the fusion of autophagosomes with lysosomes, inducing incomplete autophagy process. Intriguingly, PLP2-TM is found to associate with LC3 and Beclin1, two critical components of the autophagy pathway. These results suggest that coronavirus papain-like protease induces incomplete autophagy by interacting with Beclin1 [Chen, *et al.*, 2014].

Recent research showed that autophagy is accompanied by elevated levels of Beclin1 (BECN1). The formation of complex of BECN1 and autophagy-related genes (ATG) 14 is important for the initial nucleation steps of autophagy. Gassen, *et al.* [2019] found that MERS-CoV multiplication reduces autophagy through distinct viral proteins, which results in reduced BECN1 levels and ATG14 oligomerization, thus blocking the fusion of autophagosomes and lysosomes (Figure 3-3).

Immunopathology

Recent studies strongly indicate that virus-induced immune disorders and abnormalities play a vital role in fatal pneumonia caused by HCoV infection. A fast and well-coordinated innate immune response is the first line of defense against viral infections, but dysregulated and excessive immune responses may lead to immunopathology [Channappanavar, *et al.*, 2016; Channappanavar and Perlman, 2017].

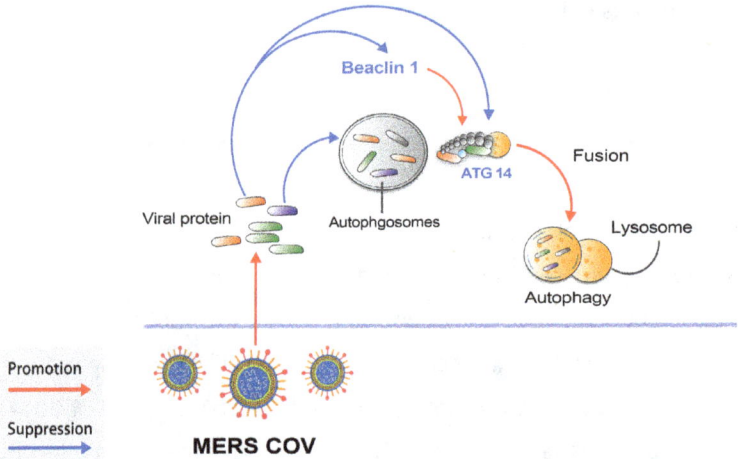

Figure 3-3 The potential mechanism by which HCoV affects autophagy.

MERS-CoV multiplication reduces autophagy through distinct viral proteins, which result in reduced BECN1 levels and ATG14 oligomerization, blocking the fusion of autophagosomes and lysosomes.

Reproduced from Gassen, et al. [2019].

Neutrophils and monocyte-macrophages are key innate immune cells that make up a large proportion of tissue infiltrating innate leukocytes following a pathogen challenge. They are rapidly recruited to the site of infection and are facilitated following the recognition of pathogen-associated molecular patterns (PAMPs) by the cell surface and endosomal toll-like receptors, leading to the activation of a cascade of signaling events, resulting in the production of antiviral molecules like interferons (IFNs), interferon-stimulated genes (ISGs), and inflammatory cytokines and chemokines. Inflammatory monocyte-macrophages and neutrophils also participate in the phagocytosis of virus-infected cells and orchestrate effective adaptive T cell responses, both of which are essential for effective virus clearance [Channappanavar, *et al.*, 2020].

The following facts highly suggest the existence and importance of immune abnormalities in severe HCoV infection:

(1)   Although most healthy individuals suffer from mild to moderate respiratory disease induced by HCoV, people with weakened immunity and comorbidities will experience severe respiratory disease and usually develop acute respiratory distress syndrome (ARDS). It has been clinically shown that MERS-CoV and COVID-19 cause severe diseases in immunocompromised and comorbid patients, in whom the activity of NK and T cells are often in "senescent" and "exhausted" status [Xu, *et al.*, 2020; Smits, *et al.*, 2010].

(2)   Viruses infect immune cells. Antigen staining shows that in addition to airway and alveolar epithelial cells and vascular endothelial cells, macrophages, monocytes, and lymphocytes are also detected in SARS-CoV and MERS-CoV virus particles and virus genomes [Nicholls, *et al.*, 2003; Gu, *et al.*, 2005]. There is evidence that macrophages infected with SARS-CoV show delayed but elevated levels of interferon and other proinflammatory cytokines [Law, *et al.*, 2005].

(3)   Peripheral blood neutrophils and monocytes increase in patients with fatal SARS, and CD4 and CD8 T cell counts decrease.

(4)   During SARS-CoV infection, dendritic cells (DC) and other PBMC-derived cells that are closely related to immunity, are also infected and show abnormal functions. The dysregulation and/or exaggeration of DC and macrophage responses to cytokines and chemokines may play an important role in the pathogenesis of SARS. DC induces low-level expression of the antiviral cytokine IFN-α/β and moderates up-regulation of pro-inflammatory cytokines TNF-α and IL-6 and significant up-regulation of inflammatory chemokines.

(5)   Infection with SARS-CoV and MERS-CoV has been accompanied with suppression of innate immune response. Coronavirus has an evolutionary strategy against the host's antiviral responses. HCoV proteins have been characterized to exhibit innate immunosuppressive effects in cellular models. As the first-line defense in the immune system, suppression of innate immune response by these HCoVs has impeded the host's ability to restrict infection. HCoV can directly or indirectly inhibit interferon (IFN) production through various mechanisms. In many infected cases, the level of type I interferon decreases. This is especially true for critically ill patients with SARS and MERS. It is also shown that SARS-CoV and MERS-CoV are capable of evading type I IFN production and signaling to different extents (Kindler, *et al.*, 2013).

(6) It is now believed that both SARS-CoV and MERS-CoV encode a variety of structural and non-structural proteins which can antagonize the IFN response. HCoV reaches high titers very early after infection and contains multiple proteins that inhibit the IFN response, suggesting that early antagonism of the IFN response may delay or evade the innate immune response. Delayed IFN signaling further coordinates the inflammatory monocyte-macrophages (IMMs) response, leading to an unregulated inflammatory response and made T cells sensitive to apoptosis [Channappanavar and Perlman, 2017].

(7) All known CoVs encode a macrodomain within the large transmembrane protein nonstructural protein 3 (nsp3). It is reported that the conserved SARS-CoV macrodomain suppresses the early IFN and proinflammatory cytokine response, not just the innate immune response, and promotes pathological changes, such as edema in the lung [Fihr, *et al.*, 2016].

(8) HCoV-specific T cells are essential for virus clearance. It is known that when the virus is infected, T cell-mediated adaptive immunity has abnormality, which may be related to DC damage and IFN production disorders.

A summary of the immunopathology to HCoV pathogenesis is demonstrated in Figure 3-4.

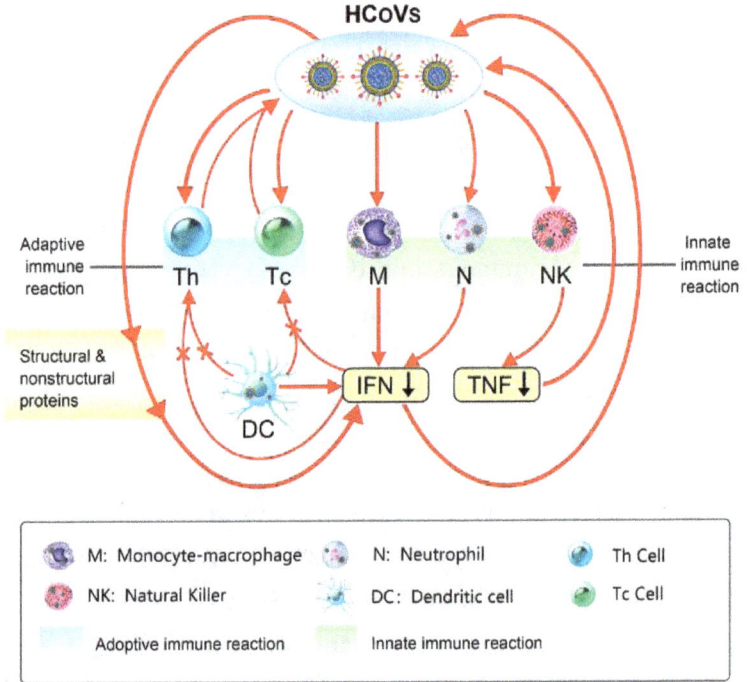

Figure 3-4 A summary of causes and consequences of cytokine storm and immunopathology to HCoV pathogenesis.

HCoV: human coronaviruses; ALI: acute lung injury; ARDS: acute respiratory distress syndrome. From Channappanavar and Perlman [2017].

Fibrosis

During SARS-CoV infection, bronchial epithelial exfoliation, cilia loss, multinucleated syncytium cells, and squamous metaplasia are often shown on lung pathology. Monocytes/macrophages and neutrophils migrate into the lungs through endothelial cells that trigger pulmonary fibrosis [Gu and Korteweg, 2007]. It has been reported that nearly 20% of SARS patients develop pulmonary fibrosis within 9 months of infection [Tse, *et al.*, 2004]. Nicholls, *et al.* [2003] found that fibrosis appears in the lungs at the same time as inflammation infiltration 10 days after the onset of SARS.

It has been shown that TGF-β1 is elevated in plasma and lung tissues in the early stages of SARS patients [Lee, *et al.*, 2004; Beijing Group of National Research Project for SARS, 2013]. TGF-β1 is the

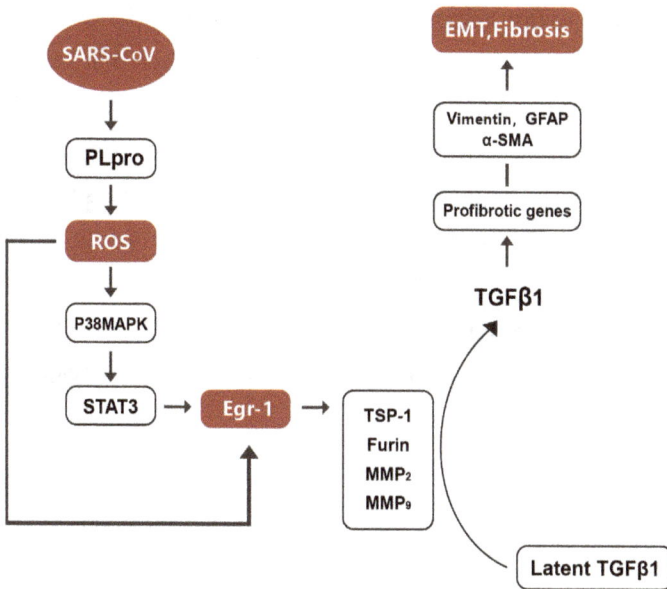

Figure 3-5 The mechanism of pulmonary pro-fibrosis induced by SARS-CoV.

SARS-CoV PLpro induces the TGF-β1-mediated profibrotic response via ROS/p38MAPK/ STAT3/Egr-1. ROS also directly up-regulates Egr-1. Biologically active TGF-β1 induces epithelial-mesenchymal transition (EMT) and fibrosis through up-regulation of several profibrotic genes.

MMP-2: matrix metalloproteinase 2; MMP-9: matrix metalloproteinase 9.

Reproduced from Li, et al. [2016].

main mediator of fibrosis [Rogel, *et al.*, 2011]. A series of transcription factors can activate the TGF-β1 promoter, which is regulated by various cellular kinases. It is reported that latent TGF-β1 in the extracellular matrix is proteolytically converted by proprotein-converting enzymes [furin, thrombospondin 1 (TSP-1), matrix metalloproteinase 2 (MMP-2), and MMP-9] into biologically active TGF-β1 [Kim, *et al.*, 2007].

SARS-CoV has a papain-like proteases (PLpro), which regulates the innate immune response and participates in SARS-CoV-induced pulmonary fibrosis. Research by Li, *et al.* [2016] showed that SARS-CoV PLpro triggers the production of TGF-β1 through the ROS/p38MAPK/STAT3/Egr-1 pathway. ROS also can directly up-regulate Egr-1. TGF-β1 mediates the up-regulation of profibrotic genes such as vimentin, GFAP, and α-SMA, and then promotes epithelial-mesenchymal transition (EMT) and fibrosis.

The mechanism of SARS CoV-induced pulmonary fibrosis is very complicated. The results of various studies are summarized in Figure 3-5.

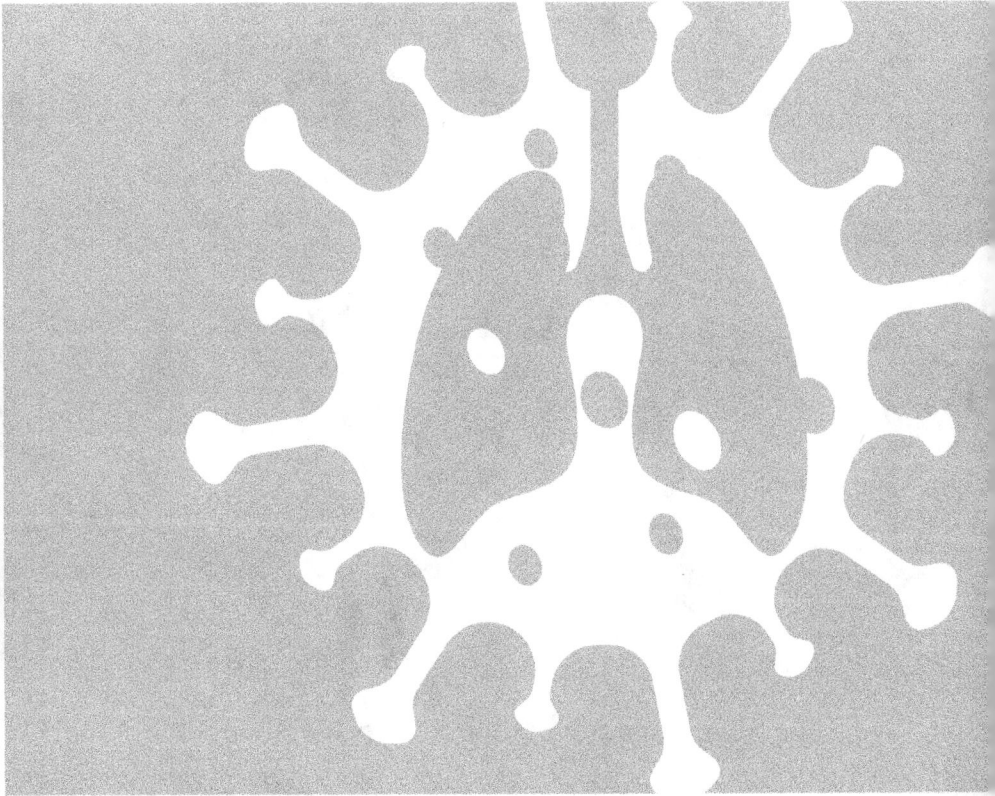

Oxidative Stress and ROS During Viral Respiratory Infections

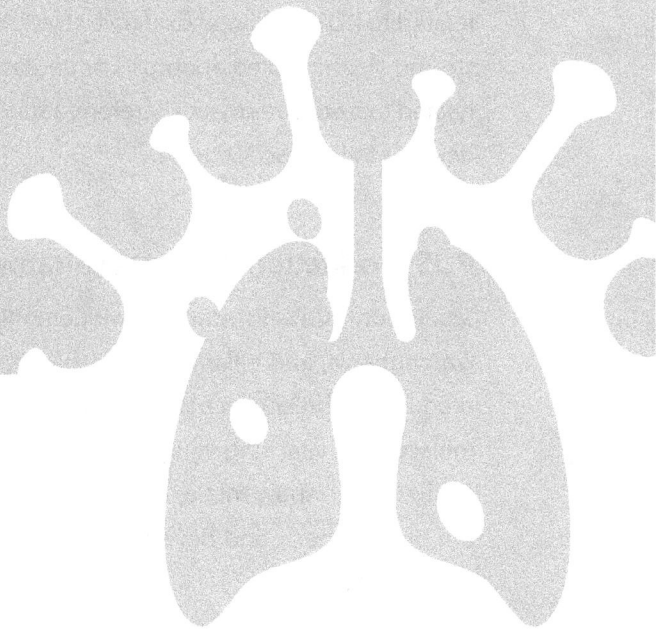

Oxidative stress

Oxidative stress means an imbalance between oxidants and antioxidants in favor of the oxidants, leading to a disruption of redox signaling and control and/or molecular damage [Sies, 2015]. Reactive oxygen species (ROS) is main cause of oxidative stress. Virus-induced oxidative stress plays a critical role in the viral life cycle as well as the pathogenesis of viral injury. Also, in response to ROS generation by a virus, a host cell activates an antioxidative defense system for its own protection.

In the previous chapter, the pathogenic effect of ROS has been discussed in many places. However, because this toxic free radical is not only closely related to the incidence of HCoV infection, the main therapeutic effect of hydrogen introduced in this book is mainly related to ROS-mediated oxidative stress. In fact, whether cytokine storms, virus-induced apoptosis or necrosis, or fibrosis, all may be related to oxidative stress. Therefore, a special chapter is specifically devoted to its description.

ROS production during respiratory viral infections

Studies on HCoVs infections have demonstrated that pneumonia, lymphopenia, and inflammatory cell infiltration are parallel to the production of ROS, which is considered to be the primary pathogenic molecules of viral lung injury [Vlahos, *et al.*, 2012]. There are several studies which show that oxidative stress plays an important role in the pathogenesis and development of viral infections [Khomich, *et al.*, 2018].

Apart from HCoVs, respiratory viruses which cause infections of the upper or lower respiratory tract comprises influenza (IV), human respiratory syncytial (HRSV), human rhino (HRV), human metapneumo (HMPV), and parainfluenza. Many of them cause common clinical syndromes, have similar pathological mechanisms that cause lung damage, so this chapter intends to introduce the research progress of oxidative stress during respiratory viral infections.

All respiratory viral infections are accompanied by clear evidence of increased ROS production. Increased levels of ROS and increased levels of nitric oxide synthase 2 (iNOS) and nitrosotyrosine have been reported in the lung tissues of patients who died in the fatal influenza virus (IV) infection pandemic. According to reports, oxidative products, such as DNA product 8-hydroxydeoxyguanosine, lipid product malondialdehyde, F2-isoprostaglandin, 7-ketocholesterol, and 7β-hydroxycholesterol were detected in plasma and urine of patients with influenza virus infection. The content of carbonyl groups in both protein and protein products increased significantly [Ng, *et al.*, 2014]. Not only during IV infection but also three months after virus clearance, elevated levels of sterol oxidation products were detected [Ng, *et al.*, 2014]. IV-infected mice and cell lines also exhibited enhanced ROS production and destruction of antioxidant defense capabilities.

Other respiratory viruses also promote the production of ROS. Human respiratory syncytial virus (HRSV) [Casola, *et al.*, 2001] and Sendai virus (SeV) [Gao, *et al.*, 2016; Qian, *et al.*, 2019] trigger an increase in total ROS levels in airway cells. It has been reported that in infants with acute bronchiolitis induced by HRSV, plasma lipid peroxidation products and oxidized glutathione (GSH) levels are increased. A decrease in antioxidant capacity is detected in the cells of infants and mice infected with HRSV, which also suggests the presence of oxidative stress [Hosakote, *et al.*, 2011]. It has been reported that the levels of antioxidant enzymes in the airway cells of mice infected with human HMPV have been reduced [Bao, *et al.*, 2008]. Studies have shown that HRV induces the production of ROS in airway cells by increasing the production of $O_2 \bullet^-$.

Lin, *et al.* [2016] demonstrated that acute lung injury caused by H5N1 infection is due to excessive ROS production which may trigger oxidized phospholipid signaling and cause acute lung injury through the TLR4-TRIF-TRAF6 cascade [Brydon, *et al.*, 2005]. To, *et al.* [2014] used immunofluorescence technology to prove that influenza A virus will enter alveolar macrophages within one hour after infection, and promote the significant enhancement of Nox2 oxidase-dependent oxidation activity in macrophages, which release a large amount of ROS. Perrone, *et al.* [2008] used flow cytometry to quantify the cellular immune response of mouse lung infections and demonstrated that macrophages and neutrophils aggregate in the lungs of highly pathogenic H1N1 and H5N1 influenza virus-infected mice. These cells release ROS and reactive species, such as $\bullet OH$ and $ONOO^-$, the excessive production of which promotes the release of a large number of pro-inflammatory factors, triggering inflammation. The inflammatory cells produce ROS again, forming a vicious cycle. Selemidis, *et al.* [2013] showed that influenza A virus infects alveolar macrophages in the respiratory tract, leading to the activation of

Toll-like receptor 7 (TLR7), which generates a large amount of ROS through NADPH oxidase containing Nox2.

Source of ROS in airway epithelial cells of virus infection

Respiratory viruses are known to induce ROS-producing enzymes, including nicotinamide adenine dinucleotide phosphate oxidase (NADPH oxidase, Nox) and xanthine oxidase (XO), and destroy the defense capacity of antioxidants (Figure 4-1). The increased activity

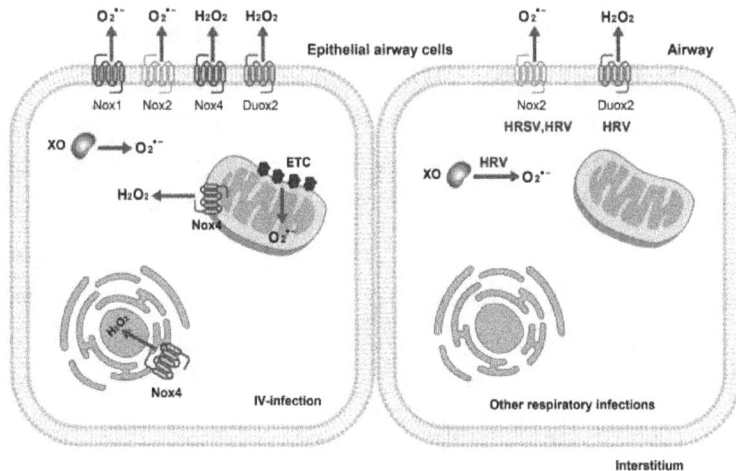

Figure 4-1 Production of ROS in airway epithelial cells infected with influenza virus or human respiratory syncytial virus (HRSV) and rhinovirus.

The sources are mainly represented by nicotinamide adenine dinucleotide phosphate oxidases (NADPH oxidases, Nox), Dual oxidase (Duox) and xanthine oxidase (XO).

XO: xanthine oxidase; ETC: electron transport chain.

Modified from Khomich, et al. [2018].

of the Nox and Dual oxidase (Duox) families is observed both in *vivo* and *in vitro* [Amatore, *et al.*, 2015; Altenhofer, *et al.*, 2015].

(1) Nox2 is a phagozyme. IV, HRSV, HRV, and SeV viruses induce generation of ROS through Nox2 after infection *in vitro* and *in vivo* [Ye, *et al.*, 2015; Fink, *et al.*, 2008]. It has been reported that respiratory RNA viruses induce Nox2-mediated ROS production in the endosomes of alveolar macrophages. In addition, the recruitment of neutrophils and monocytes from the blood to the infection site may significantly promote the superoxide anion produced by Nox2 during the infection process of influenza and HRSV.

(2) Nox4, another NADPH oxidase, has been shown to be involved in the production of ROS in IV-infected lung cancer cells or major airway epithelial cells. The survival period of IV-infected mice with inactivated Nox1 is prolonged, which indicates that Nox1 is a harmful source of ROS [Selemidis, *et al.*, 2013]. In polarized airway epithelial cells infected with HRV, Nox1-derived ROS is responsible for triggering barrier dysfunction, which will be introduced later.

(3) Duox2, belonging to the Nox/Duox family, is proved to be another source of ROS during IV infection [Fink, *et al.*, 2008; Grandvaux, *et al.*, 2015]. Duox2 activity is clearly induced

during IV infection *in vitro* and *in vivo*. The high activity of Duox2 in primary tracheobronchial epithelial cells of humans infected with HRV is reported.

(4) Xanthine oxidase, which is involved in the catabolism of purine nucleic acid bases, catalyzing the conversion of hypoxanthine to xanthine and further to uric acid, is known to be another IV-induced ROS producing enzyme. Increased levels of XO are observed in the serum, lung tissue, and bronchoalveolar lavage fluid of IV-infected mice [Akaike, *et al.*, 1990].

(5) Mitochondria. IV are known to cause electrons to leak from the respiratory chain, suggesting that mitochondria is an important source of ROS in the viral infections. The production of ROS in mitochondria may be mediated by Duox2 or Nox2, both of which have been shown to induce mitochondrial dysfunction [Dikalov, *et al.*, 2011; Daiber, *et al.*, 2017].

Compared with viruses such as human immunodeficiency virus (HIV) and hepatitis B and C viruses (HBV and HCV), the data about molecular mechanisms by which respiratory viruses induce large amounts of ROS production and its pathogenesis is still lacking. It is suggested that overexpression of proton channel protein M2 activates protein kinase C (PKC) and increases ROS production [Lazrak, *et al.*, 2009]. Also, it has been reported that SARS-CoV can produce a 3CL-Pro (protease) protein, which can induce the production of ROS and NFκB activation [Lin, *et al.*, 2017].

Role of respiratory viruses in resisting oxidative defense pathways

Respiratory viruses not only increase the production of ROS, but also affect the cellular defense system against ROS. The antioxidant defense system is composed of a variety of enzymes, transcription factors, and a series of low molecular weight molecules commonly known as antioxidants, which mainly involves the direct removal of ROS, defensing enzyme circulation or regulation of redox sensitive transcription factors.

The key transcription factor controlling the expression of a series of defense enzymes is nuclear factor E2 related factor 2 (Nrf2) [Nguyan, *et al.*, 2009]. This has been mentioned in many places in the introduction of the previous chapters. During normal levels of ROS production, Nrf2 is retained in the cytoplasm by algae-like ECH-related protein 1 (Keap1). When ROS production increases, Nrf2 dissociates from Keap1 and transfers to the nucleus, where Nrf2 binds to the antioxidant response element (ARE) [Kwak, *et al.*, 2002]. The Nrf2 gene itself also contains ARE-like sequences in its promoter. Among the target genes regulated by Nrf2 are superoxide dismutase, catalase, peroxidase, and glutathione peroxidase. HRSV reduces mRNA levels and Nrf2 levels in the airway epithelial nucleus [Hosakote, *et al.*, 2009]. Further research found that HRSV can induce the deacetylation of Nrf2 and subsequent degradation of the

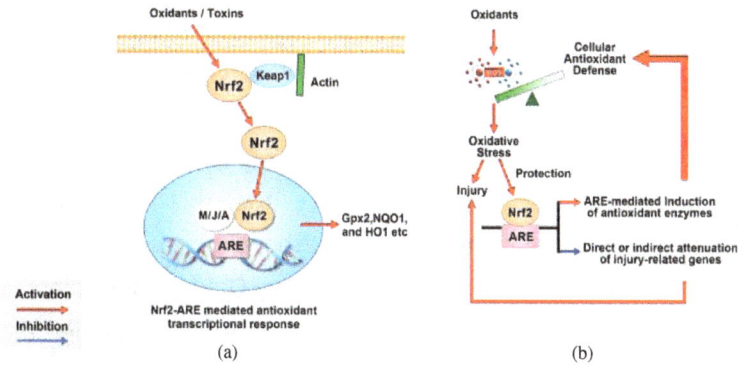

Figure 4-2 NF-E2-related factor 2 (Nrf2)-dependent antioxidant mechanism.

(a) Nrf2 dissociates from Kelch-like ECH-associated protein 1 (Keap1) on exposure to oxidants and translocates to the nucleus where it binds to the promoter region of antioxidant enzymes containing antioxidant response element (ARE) such as Gpx2, NQO1, and GCLC, HO-1. (b) Nrf2-dependent effector mechanism involves transcription of antioxidant enzymes and attenuation of injury-related genes that provide protection against oxidant-induced acute lung injury.

Reproduced from Mittal, et al. [2014].

proteasome, resulting in the down-regulation of antioxidant enzyme expression (Figure 4-2).

Effect of ROS on respiratory virus life cycle

Does ROS have a direct effect on the respiratory virus life cycle; is it a promotion effect on the replication of virus itself? Research in this area is very scarce. It is suggested that ROS is a proliferation medium and can promote virus replication in cells [To, *et al.*, 2014]. Some people think that ROS-induced cell death and lysis can promote the release and spread of virions, thereby stimulating the replication of those respiratory viruses with a lytic life cycle. Nrf2 overexpression negatively affects the replication of influenza virus, while knockdown leads to increased virus entry and replication.

There is evidence that ROS enhances the pathogenesis of infections such as influenza [Peterhans, 1997; Levander, 1997]. Studies on mice infected with influenza virus have shown that 5 or 6 days after death, cells extracted from the dead mice show higher levels of O_2^- and xanthine oxidase (an enzyme that synthesizes O_2^-), indicating that the generation of ROS has increased [Hennet, et al., 1992]. In addition, the concentration of antioxidants generally decreases during infection.

According to reports, during the HRV life cycle, ROS stimulates the expression of intercellular adhesion molecule 1 (ICAM1), which is the main receptor for the entry of the virus. Consistent with this, treatment to reduce glutathione (GSH) reduces virus-mediated ICAM1 activation. The content of GSH in SeV-infected cells is significantly reduced [Nencioni, et al., 2003]. Supplementation of exogenous GSH will inhibit virus replication [Palamara, et al., 1996], while on the contrary, depletion will increase virus titer.

Further research shows that influenza virus binds with sialic acid on cells membranes through a glycoprotein called hemagglutinin (HA) [Belding, et al., 1970]. The hemagglutinin protein locates on viral surface and is synthesized in an inactive form HA and activated by specific proteases into HA1 and HA2. The cleavage of inactive form HA into HA1 and HA2 is an important determinant of influenza virulence. If the influenza virus released from the cell contains inactive HA, it will be activated by some of the proteases present in the pulmonary surfactants [Rott, et al., 1995].

Effect of ROS in pathogenesis of respiratory viral infection

ROS plays a key role in the pathogenesis of respiratory viral infections, including triggering inflammation, lung epithelial destruction, tissue damage, and in some cases, even pulmonary fibrosis. These events are mutually regulated, for example, inflammation can cause lung damage and epithelial dysfunction, and vice versa. It is known that in chronic hepatitis B and C, there is a clear correlation between the degree of oxidative stress and the severity of the disease. Similar manifestations may occur during viral lung injury.

Promote leukocyte recruitment

ROS plays a specific role in leukocyte recruitment. There is substantial evidence that the extravasation of inflammatory stimuli by leukocytes is regulated by the oxidative stress produced by leukocytes. It has been shown that the adhesion of neutrophils to the surface of endothelial cells can cause biphasic reactions related to endogenous ROS production in endothelial cells. Oxidative stress can regulate endothelial cell adhesion molecules (CAM) expression by directly activating CAM, such as vascular cell adhesion protein 1 (VCAM1), intercellular adhesion molecule 1(ICAM1), and E-selectin, and by transcription-dependent mechanisms involving redox-sensitive transcription factors (i.e., NF-κB and AP-1).

The promoter region of ICAM-1 contains binding sites for inducible redox sensitive transcription factors such as NF-κB. TNFα-induced NF-κB activation and ICAM-1 expression in endothelial cells is dependent on oxidants that are generated by the polymorphonuclear leukocyte (PMN) NADPH oxidase complex.

Trigger large amounts of pro-inflammatory cytokines

As byproducts of cellular metabolism, the mitochondrial-derived ROS (MtROS) contributes to production of pro-inflammatory cytokines IL-1β, IL-6, and TNF-α [Bulua, et al., 2011]. Notably, MtROS has been implicated in ectodomain shedding of cytokine receptor TNF receptor–1 (TNFR1) in endothelial cells, which is important for regulation of inflammatory progression. TNF-α-converting enzyme, which mediates cleavage of TNFR1, is activated by ROS [Rowlands, et al., 2011].

Another important role of MtROS has been shown in the regulation of inflammasome, which are high-molecular-weight complexes and can activate inflammatory caspases (caspase-1 and -12) and cytokines (IL-1β and IL-18) in macrophages [Martinon, et al., 2006], and are multi-protein oligomer platforms that are composed of intracellular sensors which are coupled with caspase and interleukin activating systems [Harijith, et al., 2014].

The ROS from NADPH oxidases is present in a variety of cells, especially the professional phagocytes and endothelial cells [Pendyala, 2010], which are central to the genesis of the inflammatory response [Griffith, et al., 2009].

It is discovered that viruses, including respiratory virus, promote inflammatory process through inflammasomes [Harijith, et al., 2014]. There are three different prototypes of inflammasomes: Nod-like receptor protein (NALP)1, NALP3, and IPAF. NLRP3 inflammasome is redox sensitive. The key components of NALP3 are NLRP3, apoptosis-associated speck-like protein (ASC), and caspase-1. The NLRP3 inflammasome has been shown to interact with redox-sensitive protein thioredoxin (Trx)-binding protein-2 (TBP-2). ROS serves as important inflammasome activating signals. Increased intracellular ROS generation mediates dissociation of TBP-2 from Trx, enabling association with NLRP3 inflammasome and resulting in its activation (Figure 4-3) [Zhou, et al., 2010].

There is also evidence that activation of NFκB signaling plays an important role in inflammation mediated by ROS. Respiratory viruses induce NFκB signaling *in vivo* and *in vitro* in a ROS-dependent manner. Studies have shown that IV, HRSV, and other viral infections in the body can trigger the massive production of pro-inflammatory cytokines and chemokines (such as TNFα, IL6, and IL8), called cytokine storms, which has been mentioned previously [Tisoncik, et al., 2012]. One of the key mediators for inducing cytokines and chemokines is NFκB, which is a key player in coordinating innate and inflammatory responses and lymphocyte maturation in the adaptive immune system. In IV-infected mice, NFκB activation is accompanied by increased production of cytokines such as IL6, IL8, TNFα, CCL5 / RANTES, and CXCL10 (C-X-C motif chemokine 10) [Go, et al., 2011].

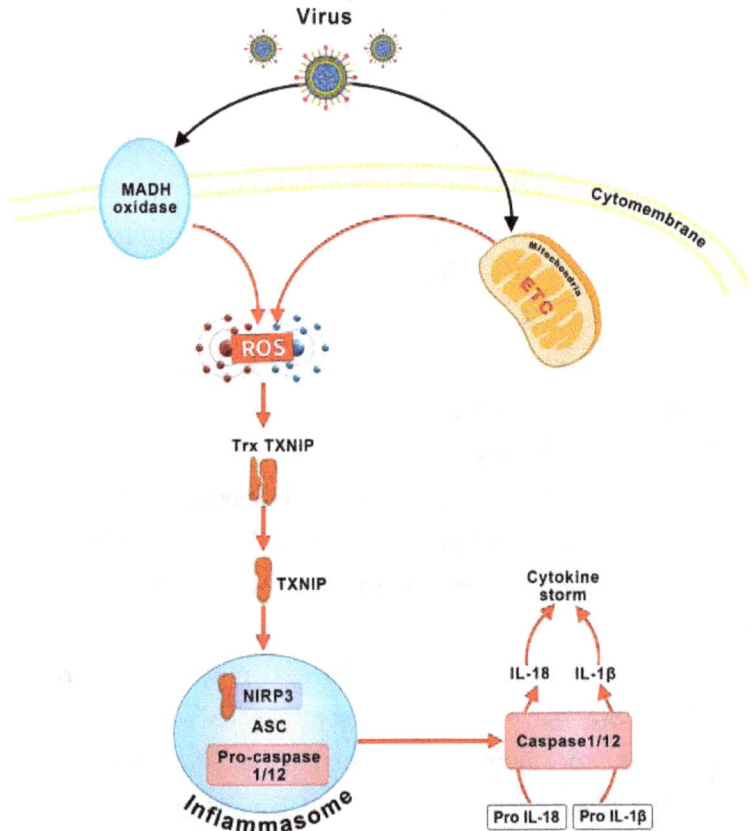

Figure 4-3   Inflammasome activation by ROS induced by viruses.

Intracellular overgeneration of ROS through NADPH oxidase or mitochondrial ETC is sensed by a complex of Trx and thioredoxin interacting protein (TXNIP), which dissociates and enables the binding of TXINP with NLRP3. This is followed by activation of NLRP3 and recruitment of apoptosis-associated speck-like protein (ASC) and pro-caspase1/12 proteins, leading to formation of active inflammasome. Active NLRP3 inflammasome cleaves pro-interleukin-1 (IL-1) beta and pro-IL-18 to active IL1 beta and IL-18, which induce cytokine storm subsequently.

ETC: Electron transport chain.

Modified from Zhou, et al. [2010].

Induce airway epithelial barrier dysfunction

Another pathological result of increased ROS production in the presence of respiratory viruses is barrier dysfunction [Comstock, et al., 2011; Unger, et al., 2014]. The vascular endothelium lining the blood vessels forms a continuous, semi-permeable restrictive barrier, allowing macromolecules, inflammatory cells, and fluid to pass between the blood and tissue spaces. There are two different transport pathways across the endothelial barrier, transcellular (transcellular) and paracellular (intercellular). Paracellular pathways are strictly controlled by interendothelial junctions (IEJs) and tight junctions (TJs), and are the main pathways for vascular leakage observed under various inflammatory conditions [Woodfin, et al., 2010].

The oxidative stress produced by leukocytes at the site of inflammation plays a key role in initiating the connection disassembly. At the site of inflammation, interepithelial junction is destroyed by several mediators released by inflammatory cells, including ROS. Most of these molecular mechanisms are focused on mediating the destruction of adherens junction (AJ) and tight junction (TJ). Oxidative stress is an inducer of actin cytoskeleton reorganization in endothelial cells, leading to junctional opening and gap formation between endothelial cells [Krizbai, et al., 2005]. Moreover, ROS is known to influence cytoskeletal dynamics by direct modification of actin and actin-associated regulatory proteins [Mittal, et al., 2014].

There is a relationship between influenza virus-induced Nox2-mediated ROS production and increased sensitivity to S. aureus pneumonia after influenza infection. HRV also disrupts the airway epithelial barrier function through ROS, thereby increasing barrier leakage and leading to increased host sensitivity to bacterial pathogens [Khomich, *et al.*, 2018].

Taken all together, it is suggested that respiratory viruses can directly invade bronchial epithelial cells or macrophages to induce ROS production. ROS can also feed back macrophages to generate more ROS. ROS can cause cell apoptosis, and through the NFκB and NLRP3 pathways, promote cytokine production. ROS and large amounts of cytokines cause abnormal structure and function of intercellular junctions (TJ and AJ). Therefore, microorganisms (such as bacteria) can enter the bloodstream through the cellular barrier that has lost function, leading to systemic infections (Figure 4-4).

Cause tissue injury

As mentioned earlier, HCoV infection can cause direct tissue damage, including apoptosis and necrosis. This consequence is also mediated through ROS.

Macrophages are evolutionary "designed" to eliminate pathogens by producing excessive oxidative stress, which, if excessive and unchecked, can lead to tissue damage. The classically activated macrophages induce tissue injury by releasing reactive oxidants including ROS that induce cell death by activation of cell death receptors, culminating in caspase activation via either an extrinsic pathway (i.e., mitochondrial independent) or an intrinsic pathway (i.e., mitochondrial dependent). In addition, oxidative stress

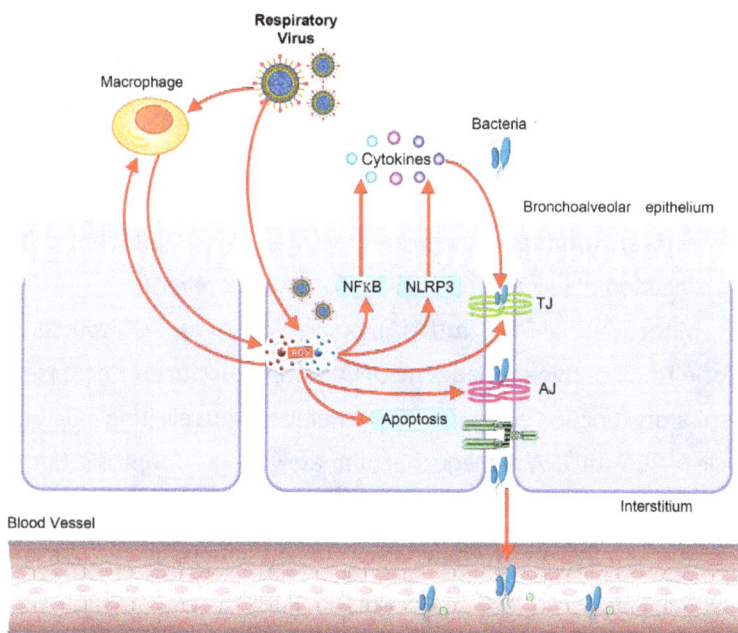

Figure 4-4   Mechanisms of destruction of the epithelial barrier caused by respiratory viruses.

Infection leads to increased ROS production, which may trigger cell death (apoptosis) and the production of cytokines by activating the NFκB pathway or by activating NLRP3 inflammatory bodies in a ROS-dependent manner, leading to inflammation and destruction of epithelial cell barrier. The destruction of the epithelial barrier leads to increased sensitivity to bacterial infections.

TJ: tight junction; AJ: adherens junction.

Reference from Khomich, et al. [2018].

produced by macrophages can induce cell death through creating an imbalance in antioxidant GSH equilibrium.

ROS are known triggers of the intrinsic apoptotic cascade. Significant mitochondrial loss of cytochrome *c* (Cyt-*c*) will lead to further ROS increase due a disrupted electron transport chain.

Normally, Cyt-c participates in shuttling electrons between Complex III and Complex IV of the mitochondrial electron transport chain; its release from the mitochondria initiates the apoptotic cascade. Enhanced ROS will significantly impact mitochondrial anion fluxes, and increase mitochondrial membrane hyperpolarization, collapse of the mitochondrial membrane potential ($\Delta\psi_m$), mitochondrial translocation of bax and Bad, and cytochrome c release.

Mitochondrial DNA (mtDNA), being close to an ROS source, is prone to oxidative damage. mtDNA damage-induced decreased respiratory function enhances ROS generation, thus eliciting a vicious cycle of ROS-mtDNA damage that ultimately trigger apoptosis [Circu, et al., 2010].

The extrinsic pathway of cell death is mediated by cell death receptors. There are four major cell death receptors, including TNF receptor 1 (TNFR1). TNF-α-induced cell death has been attributed to excessive ROS generation-sustained JNK activation and caspase activation. TNF-α is a principal pleiotropic cytokine that is secreted by activated macrophages which possesses a variety of biological properties such as production of inflammatory cytokines, cell proliferation, and cell death. Similar to TNFR1, the apoptosis induced by cell death receptor FasR has been attributed to enhanced ROS generation via NADPH oxidases and caspase activation. The enhanced ROS generation executes FasR-dependent apoptosis (Figure 4-5).

The intrinsic pathways of cell death are dependent on mitochondria-to-cytosol release of apoptogenic proteins such as Cyt-c, which trigger cell death in either a caspase-dependent or -independent manner.

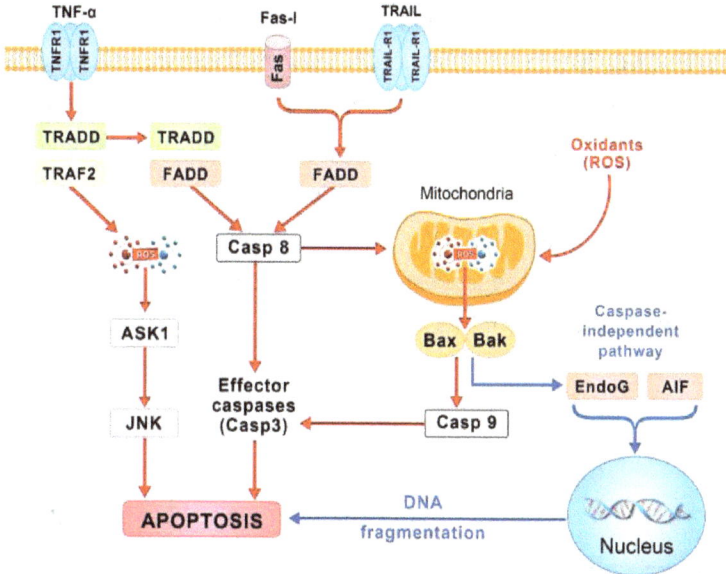

Figure 4-5   Cell apoptosis mediated by ROS and mitochondrial pathways.

For extrinsic pathway cell death, the major death receptor pathways include Fas/FasL, TNF-R1/TNFα, and TRAIL-R1/TRAIL. Binding of ligands to respective receptors activates downstream signaling and the formation of death-inducing signaling complex. At high ROS, death receptor signaling is associated with caspase-8 activation that promotes apoptosis via activation of effector caspases (e.g., caspase-3) or engages mitochondrial apoptotic signaling, leading to the release of apoptogenic factors.

For the mitochondrial intrinsic pathway, there are various apoptotic stimuli such as ROS-mediated permeabilization of the mitochondrial outer membrane and the release of pro-apoptotic proteins. Within the cytosol, the initiator procaspase-9 is recruited and activated. Caspase-9-catalyzed activation of the effector caspase-3 executes the final steps of apoptosis. In addition, mitochondrial proteins such as AIF and endoG promote caspase-independent apoptosis through nuclear translocation and mediating genomic DNA fragmentation.

ASK1: apoptosis signal-regulating kinase 1; AIF: apoptosis inducing factor; Bax/Bak: pro-apoptotic proteins; casp 8, 9: active forms of caspases-8 and -9; FADD: Fas-associated death domain; endoG: endonuclease G; FasL: Fas ligand; JNK: c-Jun N-terminal kinase; ROS: reactive oxygen species; TNF-α: tumor necrosis factor-α; TNFR1: TNF receptor-1; TRAIL: TNF-related apoptosis-inducing ligand; TRAIL-R1: Trail receptor-1; TRADD: TNF receptor-associated death domain; TRAF-2: TNF receptor-associated factor-2.

Modified from Mittal, et al. [2014].

Oxidative stress is the major trigger in Cyt-*c* release from mitochondria. The release of Cyt-*c* further enhances ROS generation from mitochondria because of uncoupling of ETC. Enhanced oxidative stress leads to oxidation of an anionic phospholipid specific to mitochondria known as cardiolipin (CL), which decreases the affinity binding with Cyt-*c*. Oxidative stress also targets oxidative modification in the inner membrane channel, hence resulting in an increase in mitochondrial permeability and Cyt-*c* release.

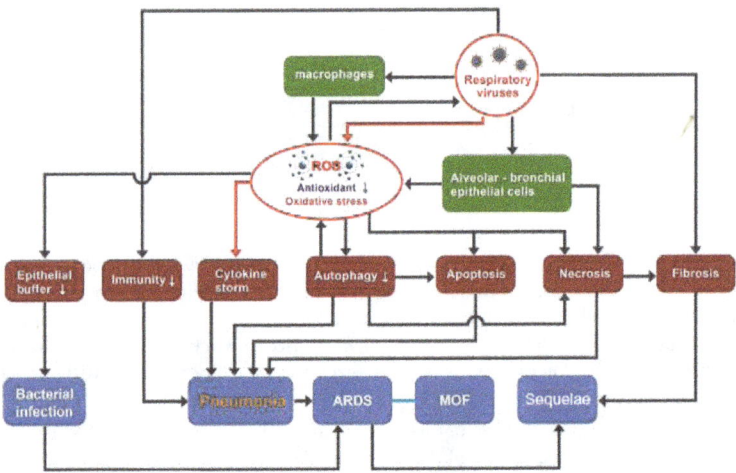

Figure 4-6 Consequences of respiratory virus infection.

The virus triggers overproduction of ROS through macrophages or through infected bronchoalveolar epithelial cells, while inhibiting antioxidant mechanisms, thereby causing oxidative stress. ROS and its induced oxidative stress can cause cytokine storms, epithelial cell apoptosis and necrosis, thereby causing pneumonia, and can further lead to acute respiratory distress syndrome and even multiple organ failure. Viruses can directly inhibit innate and adaptive immune mechanisms, leading to secondary bacterial infections and aggravating disease. Viruses can directly cause a reduction in autophagy, reduce cell protection, and can initiate the fibrosis process, causing pulmonary fibrosis, with possible sequelae.

HCoVs: human coronaviruses; ARDS: acute respiratory distress syndrome; MOF: multiple organ failure; ROS: reactive oxygen species.

Taken together, respiratory viral infections can cause different and interrelated lung damage. But most of these damages are related to ROS-mediated oxidative stress. The virus can directly pass through the infected airway epithelial cells or through macrophages, on the one hand to stimulate ROS production, on the other hand to inhibit the antioxidant mechanism, thereby causing oxidative stress. Oxidative stress mediated mainly by ROS can trigger a cytokine storm, cause acute inflammation, and promote epithelial cell apoptosis and necrosis, destroy the cell barrier, and increase secondary bacterial infections. The virus itself can suppress the body's immune function, resulting in reduced ability to clear the virus. The virus can also weaken cell autophagy and weaken cytoprotection. These factors make the condition worse, leading to ARDS and MOF. The virus also can induce fibrosis, which allows lung damage to leave sequelae (Figure 4-6).

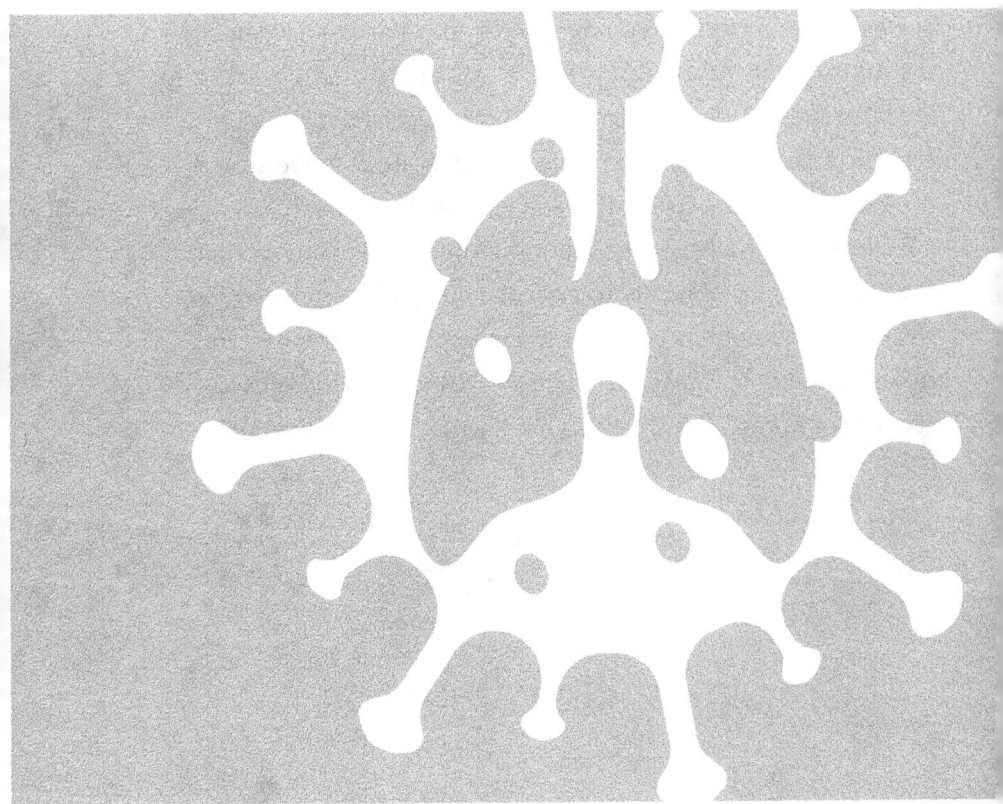

Studies on Lung Diseases with Hydrogen-Oxygen Treatment

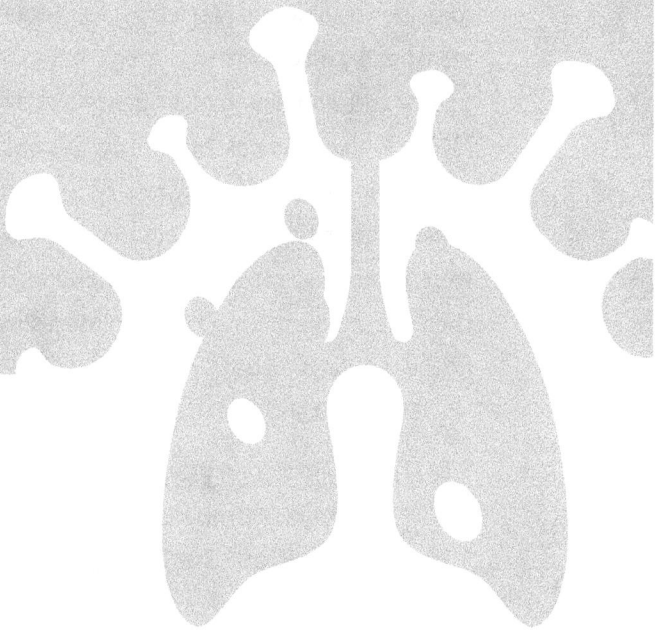

Obstructive pulmonary disease model

There is an increasing number of studies suggesting the role of oxidative stress in the development and progression of chronic obstructive pulmonary disease (COPD). There are two experimental studies on the improvement of COPD by hydrogen-oxygen inhalation.

The first study was completed by the respiratory disease team of the First Affiliated Hospital of Guangzhou Medical University [Lu, *et al.*, 2018]. It is as follows:

A COPD mouse model was established in male C57BL mice by cigarette smoke (CS) exposure. For H_2 treatment, after exposure to CS for 60 days, mice were treated with H_2 and O_2, which were generated by electrolyzing deionized water with a H_2 apparatus (provided by Shanghai Asclepius). Hydrogen (67%) and oxygen (33%) were freshly mixed with nitrogen (N_2) separated from the air, diluted to a mixture containing hydrogen (42%), oxygen (21%), and nitrogen (37%), which was passed through a rubber tube and inhaled by CS-exposed mice at a flow rate of 3.8 L/min. Each inhalation of H_2 lasted 1 hour, twice a day, at intervals of 6 to 8 hours. Control mice were placed in a closed chamber and ventilated. The animals were then subjected to lung function assessment before dissection for further analysis on day 91.

The result showed that:

(1) *H_2 inhalation attenuates CS-induced lung function decline in mice*. Compared with control mice with normal air inhalation, the CS exposed mice presented typical

COPD-like lung function decline indicated by increases in functional residual capacity (FRC), total lung capacity (TLC), Chord compliance (Cchord), forced vital capacity (FVC), and resistance index (RI), as well as a decrease in the FEV50/FVC ratio. CS-caused increases in FRC, TLC, Cchord and decrease in the FEV50/FVC were attenuated by H_2 inhalation. CS exposures significantly increased hematocrit value in blood, which was ameliorated by H_2 administration. Altogether, these results demonstrate that H_2 inhalation ameliorates CS-induced mouse lung function decline and hypoxia-induced hematocrit elevation.

(2) *H_2 inhalation attenuates CS-induced emphysema, collagen deposition in the small airway and goblet cell hypertrophy, and hyperplasia of airway epithelium.* CS-induced lung injury had a typical pathological presentation of COPD, such as damaged alveolar walls and pulmonary bullae, in mouse lungs exposed to CS. Inhalation of H_2 significantly reduced structural damage of the lung and accumulation of leukocytes in both the alveolar walls and spaces. Goblet cells from the airway epithelium of CS-exposed mice, identified by PAS staining, contained large granular stores of PAS-positive substances, which was attenuated in the H_2 treatment group. The severe collagen deposition in the small airway (50–499 μm diameter) in CS-exposed mice were reduced by H_2 inhalation (Figure 5-1).

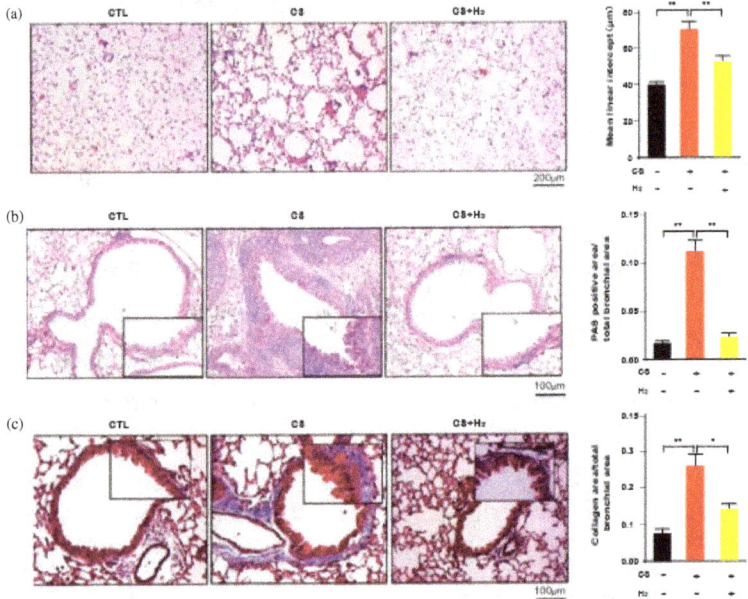

Figure 5-1 H_2 inhalation attenuates CS-induced emphysema, collagen deposition in the small airway, and goblet cell hypertrophy and hyperplasia of airway epithelium.

Comparison of H&E or Masson or PAS staining of mouse lung sections from control (CTL), CS and CS plus H_2 (CS + H_2) treated mice. Software IPP6.0 is used to assess the average linear intercept (Lm) of alveoli (a), goblet cell hyperplasia (b) and small airway remodeling (c) in at least three fields of lung section per mouse. Data is presented as mean ± SEM, n = 5 in each group. *, P < 0.05; **, P < 0.01.

From Lu, et al. [2018] with permission.

(3)   *H_2 inhalation reduces CS-induced airway inflammation and mucus hypersecretion in COPD mice.* CS exposure induced airway and lung inflammation, indicated by increases in total leukocyte number (i.e., neutrophils, macrophages, and lymphocytes) and higher levels of IL-6, TNF-α, and KC in bronchoalveolar lavage fluid (BALF). H_2 treatment attenuated these effects. The significant increased levels of Muc5ac and

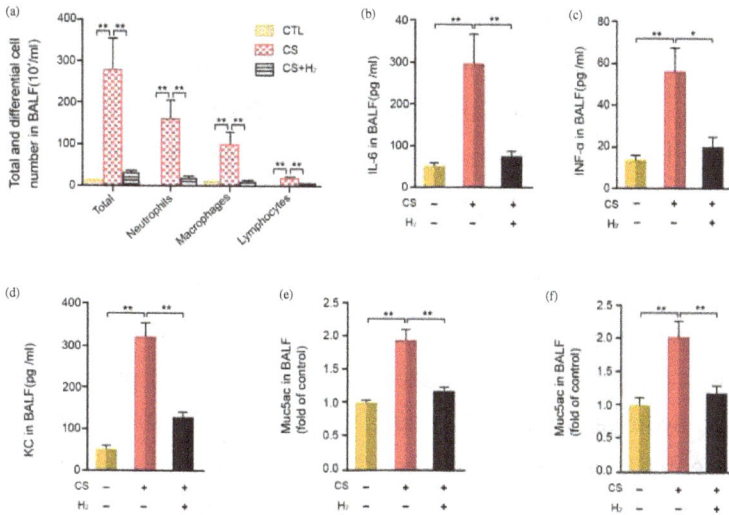

Figure 5-2 H₂ inhalation reduces CS-induced airway inflammation and mucus hypersecretion in COPD mice.

Comparison of total cell count (associated with neutrophils, macrophages, and lymphocytes) (a) and levels of IL-6 (b), TNF-α (c), and KC (d) in BALF from control (CTL), CS and CS plus H₂ (CS + H₂) treated mice. Comparison of level of Muc5ac (e) and Muc5b (f) in BALF from control (CTL), CS and CS plus H₂ (CS + H₂) treated mice. Data is presented as mean ± SEM, n = 10 in CTL group, n = 8 in CS group, n = 8 in CS + H₂ group, *, P < 0.05; **, P < 0.01.

From Lu, et al. [2018] with permission.

Muc5b in BALF from the CS-exposed group were reduced markedly by H₂ treatment (Figure 5-2). These results demonstrate that H₂ inhalation attenuates CS-induced airway inflammation and mucus hypersecretion in COPD mice.

In conclusion, these findings demonstrated that H₂ inhalation could inhibit CS-induced COPD development in mice, which is associated with reduced ERK1/2 and NF-κB-dependent inflammatory responses.

The second study was performed by a team from the First Hospital of Hebei Medical University [Liu, *et al.*, 2017], who showed that hydrogen can slow the progression of COPD-like lung disease using the same H_2 apparatus as in the previous study.

A rat COPD model was established through smoke exposure methods, and inhalation of different concentrations of hydrogen was used as the intervention. Animals were randomized into the following five groups: control group, COPD group, low-hydrogen group (Hl group), intermediate hydrogen group (Hm group), and high-hydrogen group (Hh group). Cigarette smoke and hydrogen were actually coadministered during a 4-month period. After exposure to cigarette smoke for two times every day in the 4-month period, the Hl group was given 21% O_2 + 2% H_2 by inhalation and the Hm group was given 21% O_2 + 22% H_2 by inhalation using a hydrogen atomizer and 15% O_2 + 85% N_2 at a flow rate of 1:2, whereas the Hh group was given 21% O_2 + 41.6% H_2 by inhalation with a hydrogen atomizer and 100% N_2 at a flow rate of 5:3. The rats in the control group received no intervention over the 4 months of the experimental period.

Results showed that: (1) Hydrogen administration slows weight loss in a cigarette smoke-induced rat model; (2) Hydrogen coadministration improves lung functions; and (3) Hydrogen coadministration reduces the infiltration of inflammatory cells. The number of total white blood cells, neutrophil granulocytes, and macrophages were significantly increased in the BALF of the COPD group (all $P < 0.01$). Compared with the COPD group, these cells were decreased in the Hl, Hm, and Hh groups ($P < 0.01$ or $P < 0.05$). There was no significant difference between the Hm and Hh groups in these cell numbers. (4) Hydrogen coadministration ameliorates pathologic changes of lung in a cigarette smoke-induced rat model. The alveolar ducts, alveolar sacs, and pulmonary alveoli of rats in the COPD group were significantly expanded; the alveoli were structurally disordered, the alveolar wall showed signs of thinning and breaking, and some had fused into bullae. The ciliated cells showed degeneration and necrosis. The pulmonary artery wall was thickened, and the lumen narrowed, with varying degrees of peripheral neutrophil, lymphocyte, and mononuclear macrophage infiltration. The lungs in rats of the Hl, Hm, and Hh groups were slightly reduced compared to those of rats in the COPD group, and the appearance of the lungs was also improved. The pulmonary artery walls showed mild thickening; the alveolar wall was relatively thin, inflammatory cells were decreased, and the fracture conditions were improved, compared with those in the COPD group.

What is different from the first study is that the second study observed hydrogen effect on ultrastructural changes of lung in a rat model [Liu, et al., 2017].

SEM observations showed alveolar septa with a smooth surface with no fracture in the control group. Compared with the control group, the alveolar septum in the COPD group was thinner and showed subsequent fracture. The structural integrity of the alveolar wall was damaged, and the alveolar epithelial cells were disorganized. Alveolar hyperinflation occurred, and lymphocytes and cell shed debris were present in the alveoli. The alveolar septum was thinner, occasionally ruptured, and there were a few inflammatory cells in the HI group. The alveolar septum showed a smooth surface in the Hm and Hh groups, and no fracture was present. The alveolar wall showed structural integrity and the alveolar epithelial cells were arranged in an orderly manner. There was no alveolar bleeding or exudation, and only occasional inflammatory cell infiltration was seen. Thus, the alveolar condition was improved in the Hm and Hh groups, compared to the HI group.

The ultrastructural changes of alveolar type II epithelial cells under TEM showed that the microvilli on the surface of alveolar type II epithelial cells were uncompromised in the control group, the cristae and membrane of mitochondria showed a clear structure, the rough endoplasmic reticulum was regular in structure, and the nucleus had clear boundaries. Compared with the control group, the microvilli on the surface of alveolar type II epithelial cells were reduced in the COPD group, the cristae and membrane of the mitochondria were markedly fused, and giant mitochondria were visible. The rough endoplasmic reticulum was expanded and the perinuclear gap was widened. However, in the HI, Hm, and Hh groups, these showed significant improvement (Figure 5-3).

The second study [Liu, et al., 2017], with immunohistochemical staining, discovered that hydrogen coadministration reduces the mRNA and protein expression of TNF-α, IL-6, IL-17, IL-23, MMP-12, caspase-3, and caspase-8, but increases TIMP-1 expression, as shown in Figure 5-4.

As stated above, in this study, cigarette smoke exposure was used to establish COPD-like lung disease model in rats. These rats exhibited typical pathologic changes of COPD that were accompanied with decreased lung function. It was found that hydrogen inhalation

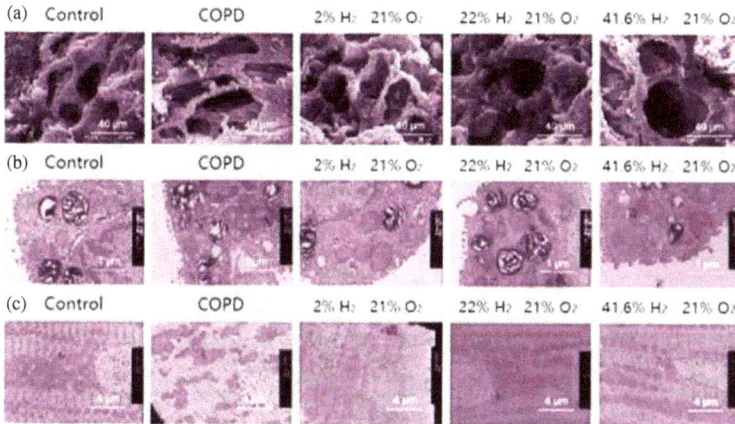

Figure 5-3 Effect of hydrogen on changes in the ultrastructure of COPD-like lung disease rats.

(a) Lung tissue observation of five groups under SEM. (b) Lung tissue observation of five groups under TEM. See text for details.

COPD: chronic obstructive pulmonary disease; SEM: scanning electron microscope; TEM: transmission electron microscope.

From Liu, et al. [2017] with permission.

improves the lung pathology and function through inhibition of pulmonary inflammatory cytokines and apoptotic proteins and restoration of protease/antiprotease balance. It is suggested that hydrogen inhalation slows the development of COPD-like lung disease in a cigarette smoke-induced rat model. Higher concentrations of hydrogen may represent a more effective way.

Airway stenosis

Improving the obstruction of airways, especially small airways, and reducing airway resistance are of great significance in clinical practice of respiratory disease. Oxygen therapy and noninvasive mechanical

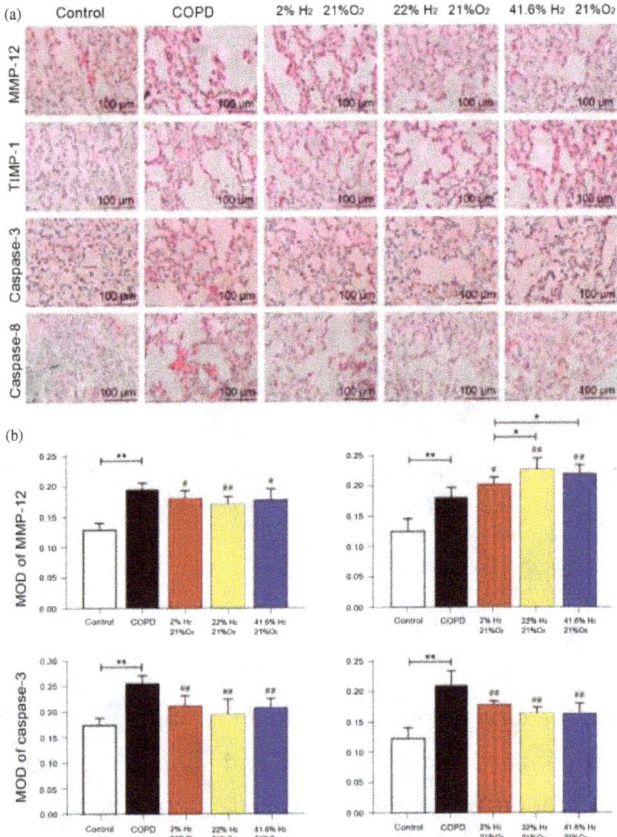

Figure 5-4 Effect of hydrogen on the expression of MMP-12, TIMP-1, caspase-3, and caspase-8 in the lung obtained from COPD-like lung disease rats, found by immunohistochemical staining.

(a) Immunohistochemical staining of the lung sections for MMP-12, TIMP-1, caspase-3, and caspase-8. (b) Quantitative analysis of the expression of MMP-12, TIMP-1, caspase-3, and caspase-8 in the lung of COPD-like lung disease rats. (n = 10 for each group; #P < 0.05, ##P < 0.01 compared with COPD group; *P < 0.05, **P < 0.01). Each experiment is repeated three times and similar results are obtained.

COPD: chronic obstructive pulmonary disease; MMP: matrix metalloproteinase; MOD: mean optical density; TIMP: tissue inhibitor of metalloproteinase.

From Liu, et al. [2017] with permission.

ventilation have limited effects on emergency management of tracheal stenosis. Low-density and low-molecular-weight gaseous helium (He) has been shown to reduce airway resistance and reduce the inspiratory power of patients with upper airway obstruction. To date, there has been no way to satisfactorily reduce the inspiratory force other than helium inhalation during emergency treatment of tracheal stenosis.

In the First Affiliated Hospital of Guangzhou Medical University, Guangzhou, China, the State Key Laboratory of Respiratory Disease team did a pioneering study showing that hydrogen inhalation could effectively reduce the resistance of tracheal stenosis, and reduce the patient's inspiratory effort [Zhou, *et al.*, 2018]. It is as follows:

Study Design: This was a prospective, single-blind, and self-control study. The primary endpoint was the patient's inspiratory effort, as assessed with a diaphragm electromyogram (EMGdi). Secondary endpoints were the transdiaphragmatic pressure (Pdi), vital signs, Borg score, and impulse oscillometry (IOS) during gas inhalation. 35 consecutive patients with tracheal stenosis were enrolled from November 2016 to June 2017. The inclusion criteria were as follows: (A) dyspnea within the previous four weeks; (B) Borg score >2 on admission; and (C) ≥ grade III stenosis. The exclusion criteria were as follows: (A) comorbidities, such as COPD, asthma, vocal insufficiency, or ventricular dysfunction, that could lead to dyspnea; (B) unable to tolerate study measurements due to severe dyspnea; and (C) no dyspnea.

Generation and Inhalation of Gas Mixtures: The medical Hydrogen-Oxygen Atomizer (AMS-H-01, provided by Shanghai Asclepius) approved by the State Food and Drug Administration was used. The machine provided an output for the mixture gas comprising 33% O_2 and 67% H_2 of 6 L per minute by electrolysis of pure water. The gas mixture was delivered to the patient through a nasal cannula.

Hydrogen Inhalation: Patients inhaled air, H_2-O_2 (H:O = 67%:33%, 6 L/min) and O_2 (3 L/min), through nasal cannula; H_2-O_2 was included in the regimen twice. The study included 4 breathing steps: (1) air for 15 min; (2) H_2-O_2 for 15 min (H_2-O_2–1); (3) O_2 for 15 min; and (4) H_2-O_2 a second time for 120 min (H_2-O_2–2). Patients breathed air for 30 min as the washout period after each breathing step. The duration of first 3 periods was set to 15 min each.

Baseline Characteristics: Among 35 patients with tracheal stenosis enrolled, 14 patients had post-intubation or tracheotomy stenosis, 4 had post-tuberculosis stenosis, and 17 had malignant stenosis. Sixteen of the 35 patients (Surface Group) who could not tolerate or refused to swallow the esophageal catheter received the noninvasive surface EMG test instead. The other 19 patients (Esophageal Group) tolerated the esophageal catheter well. Twenty-one of the 35 patients did not tolerate or refused an IOS test, and the other 14 patients underwent IOS tests.

Results showed that:

(1) *Variability of EMGdi during gas mixture inhalation*: The EMGdi decreased significantly, as did the transdiaphragmatic

pressure, when breathing H_2-O_2. In the Surface Group, the sEMGdi of the left side was significantly lower with H_2-O_2–1 than with air or O_2. A significant reduction in the sEMGdi of the right side was observed with H_2-O_2–1. In the Esophageal Group, a significant decrease in the EMGdi was observed with H_2-O_2–1. Among the 35 patients, no difference was observed between H_2-O_2–1 and H_2-O_2–2 or between air and O_2. The EMGdi decreased rapidly over 5 min after breathing H_2-O_2 and tended to be stable for 120 min. The trends in the variability of the EMGdi over time are shown in Figure 5-5.

(2) *Correlation between diaphragmatic function and stenosis percentage*: For the 16 patients in the Surface Group, delta-surface EMGdi (ΔsEMGdi) in both the left and right sides was significantly correlated with the stenosis percentage. For the 19 patients in the Esophageal Group,

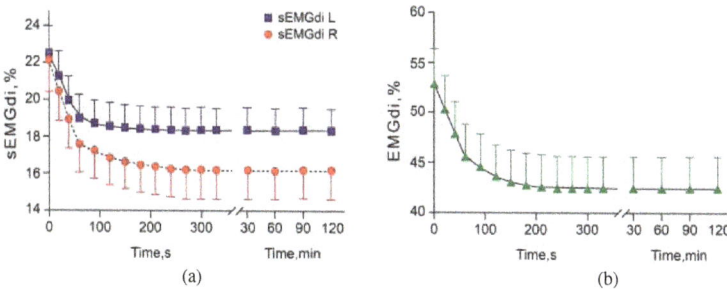

Figure 5-5 (a) Trends in the variability of left and right sEMGdi of 16 patients over time. (b) Trends in the variability of EMGdi of 19 patients over time.

From Zhou, et al. [2018] with permission.

a significant correlation between ΔEMGdi and the stenosis percentage was evident.

(3) *Correlation between diaphragmatic function and Borg score*: In the Surface Group, ΔsEMGdi in both the left and right sides was correlated significantly with the Borg scores. In the Esophageal Group, a significant correlation was evident between ΔEMGdi and Borg scores.

(4) *Pdi, vital signs, Borg score, and airway resistance*: In the Esophageal Group, a significant decrease in the Pdi was observed with H_2-O_2-1 compared with air or O_2. No difference existed between H_2-O_2-1 and H_2-O_2-2 or between air and O_2. None of the vital signs differed significantly among the 4 breathing steps.

31 patients exhibited a decrease in the Borg score. The mean reduction in the Borg score under H_2-O_2-1 was 2.02 ± 0.86 points. The Borg score significantly decreased during two H_2-O_2 inhalation steps compared with air and O_2. No difference existed between H_2-O_2-1 and H_2-O_2-2 or between air and O_2.

The IOS was performed on 14 patients successfully. While breathing H_2-O_2, R5 and R20 decreased, whereas R5-R20 did not change.

Comment

This study may be the first to pioneer the effects of a H_2-O_2 mixture in the emergency management of tracheal stenosis. When breathing H_2-O_2, the patient's diaphragmatic function, Borg score, and IOS parameters were significantly improved. These findings indicate that breathing the H_2-O_2 mixture could reduce airway resistance and decrease inspiratory effort.

Several studies have reported the use of He-O_2 mixtures in patients with upper airway obstruction [Fleming, et al., 1992; Bo, et al., 2018; Skrinskas, et al., 1983; Jaber, et al., 2001]. There was a study that showed that when breathing He-O_2, the average decrease in Pdi was 19% and 30% on the left and right, respectively. In this study, the average reductions in sEMGdi on the left and right were 18.3% and 26.5%, respectively. The mean reduction in the EMGdi in the Esophageal Group was 20.0%, and that in the Pdi was 17.6% while breathing H_2-O_2, compared to air or O_2. The effect of H_2-O_2 was similar to that of He-O_2.

According to Graham's law, the rate of gas diffusion is inversely proportional to the square root of its density. The mixture of hydrogen and oxygen in a ratio of 2:1 and has a molecular weight much smaller than air and pure oxygen. The molecular weight of air is about 29, pure oxygen is 32, and the hydrogen-oxygen mixture is about 11.88. Therefore, compared with air, the hydrogen-oxygen mixture has a lower density and a faster diffusion speed [Glauser, et al., 1969]. This may be the reason why inhalation of hydrogen and oxygen can improve airway resistance.

Asthma model

There are two studies focusing on the effect of hydrogen inhalation on asthma animal models.

The first was performed by a team from the Department of Naval Aeromedicine, the Second Military Medical University, Shanghai, China [Zhang, *et al.*, 2018].

An ovalbumin (OVA)-induced mouse model of allergic airway inflammation was established. Mice were sensitized to ovalbumin and received the mixed gas consisting of 67% H_2 and 33% O_2 produced by the AMS-H-01 Hydrogen-Oxygen Atomizer (provided by Shanghai Asclepius). The mice were placed into a transparent closed box into which the mixed gas was introduced at a rate of 200 ml/min throughout the experiment.

Results showed that:

(1)   *Hydrogen gas inhalation decreases lung resistance in the asthmatic mice model.* Lung resistance (RL) increased in the asthmatic mouse model compared with the control group and was significantly lower in the asthma-hydrogen (AH) group compared with the asthma (A) group. There was no significant difference in the respiratory rate (RR), peak flow rate (PEF), and dynamic compliance (Cdyn) among the four groups.

(2)   *Hydrogen gas inhalation improves the histology and mucus production in the asthmatic mouse model.* Mouse models exhibited cardinal histopathological signs of human asthmatic lungs, including peribronchial and perivascular inflammatory infiltrates, with most notably eosinophilia, goblet cell hyperplasia, airway wall thickening, and airway obstruction compared with the control group. Hydrogen gas inhalation attenuated this accumulation of

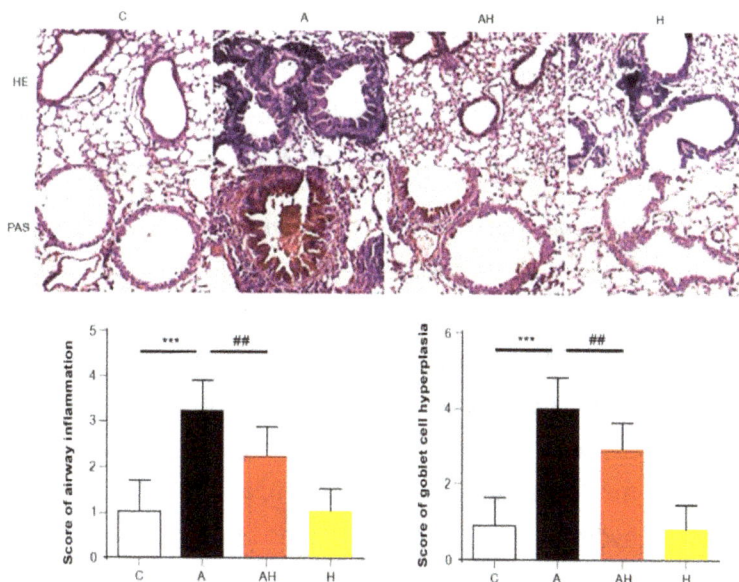

Figure 5-6 Morphologic findings and scores of bronchial wall in control animals (C, n = 10), asthmatic mice model (A, n = 10) and asthmatic mice model with hydrogen gas inhalation (AH, n = 10) and control animals with hydrogen gas inhalation (H, n = 10).

Staining with haematoxylin-eosin (HE), periodic acid-Schiff (PAS).

From Zhang, et al. [2018] with permission.

inflammatory cells and reduced the epithelial goblet cell hyperplasia (Figure 5-6).

(3) *Hydrogen gas inhalation reduces the levels of inflammatory cells in bronchoalveolar lavage fluid (BALF) from asthmatic mice model.* There was a significant increase in the number of total cells, neutrophils, eosinophils, lymphocytes, and macrophages in BALF of asthmatic mice models compared with those of controls. Hydrogen gas inhalation resulted in significant reduction in the number of total cells,

eosinophils, and lymphocytes, and a nonsignificant decrease in the number of macrophages compared with asthmatic mouse models. The pure hydrogen gas inhalation had no effect on the BALF cell numbers.

(4) *Hydrogen gas inhalation attenuates the elevated levels of inflammatory cytokines present in BALF from the asthmatic mouse model.* There was a significant increase in IL-4, IL-5, IL-13, TNF-α, and CXCL15 in BALF of asthmatic mouse models compared with those of controls. Hydrogen-oxygen gas inhalation resulted in significant reductions in the concentrations of IL-4, TNF-α, and CXCL15. The pure hydrogen gas inhalation had no effect on the levels of inflammatory cytokines in BALF.

(5) *Hydrogen gas inhalation attenuates the oxidative stress index presented in lung homogenates from asthmatic mouse models.* The levels of malondialdehyde (MDA) and myeloperoxidase (MPO) increased significantly, and the levels of superoxide dismutase (SOD) activity, glutathione (GSH), and catalase (CAT) decreased significantly in the lung tissues of the asthmatic mouse group compared with those of controls. In contrast, a significant reduction of MDA and MPO levels and a significant increase in SOD activities were observed in the asthmatic mice with hydrogen gas inhalation group. However, the levels of GSH, CAT, and 8-hydroxydeoxyguanosine (8-OHdG) did not change significantly after hydrogen gas inhalation (Figure 5-7).

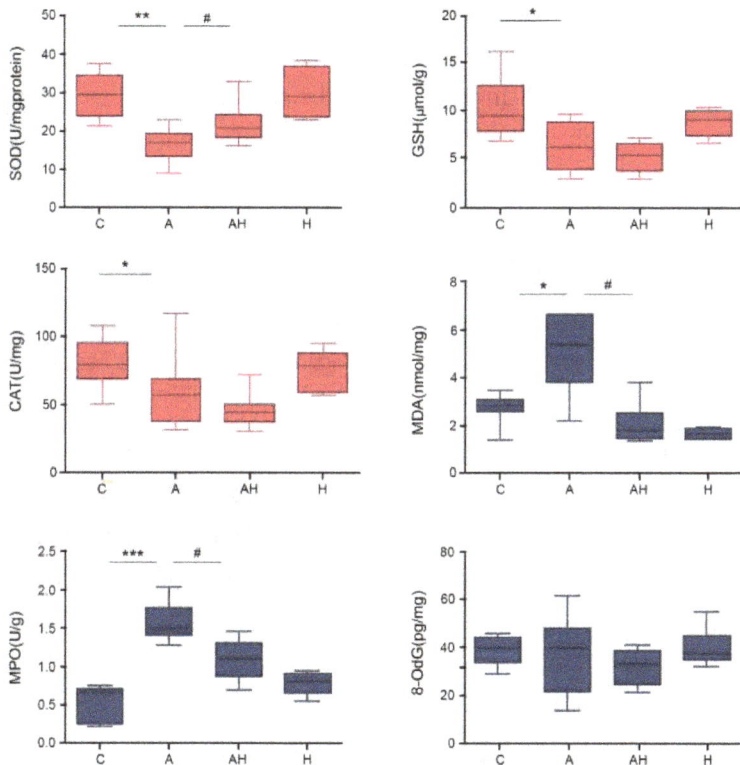

Figure 5-7 The levels or activities of SOD, MDA, GSH, CAT, MPO, and 8-OHdG of lung tissue in control animals (C, n = 10), asthmatic mouse model (A, n = 10), asthmatic mice with hydrogen gas inhalation (AH, n = 10), and control animals with hydrogen gas inhalation (H, n = 10). *P < 0.05, **P < 0.01, ***P < 0.001 compared to the control group, # P < 0.05 compared to the asthma group.

SOD: superoxide dismutase; GSH: glutathione; CAT: catalase; MDA: malondialdehyde; MPO: myeloperoxidase; 8-OHdG: 8-hydroxydeoxyguanosine.

From Zhang, et al. [2018] with permission.

The second study was conducted by the team at the State Key Laboratory of Respiratory Disease in the First Affiliated Hospital of Guangzhou Medical University, Guangzhou, China. As is known in asthma, the phagocytic capacity of alveolar macrophages is significantly reduced, which is thought to be associated with increased oxidative stress [van der Veen, *et al.*, 2020]. This study evaluated the beneficial effects of hydrogen gas inhalation on alveolar macrophage phagocytosis in an ovalbumin (OVA)-induced murine asthma model as well [Huang, *et al.*, 2019]. The test is as follows:

Female mice were intraperitoneally sensitized with aerosolized OVA. Hydrogen gas was delivered to the mice through inhalation twice a day for 7 consecutive days. Phagocytic function of alveolar macrophages isolated from bronchoalveolar lavage fluid (BALF) was assessed by fluorescence-labeled Escherichia coli as well as flow cytometry.

Results showed that the phagocytic capacity to Escherichia coli of alveolar macrophages isolated from OVA-induced asthmatic mice was decreased when compared with those of control mice, and was reversed by hydrogen gas inhalation. Hydrogen gas inhalation significantly alleviated OVA-induced airway hyperresponsiveness, inflammation, and goblet cell hyperplasia, diminished T_h2 response as well as IL-4 and IgE levels, reduced malondialdehyde (MDA) production and increased superoxide dismutase (SOD) activity. Concomitantly, hydrogen gas inhalation inhibited NF-κB activation and markedly activated Nrf2 pathway in OVA-induced asthmatic mice.

Clinical trial on acute exacerbations of chronic obstructive pulmonary disease (AECOPD)

In 2018–2019, a multicenter, randomized, parallel-controlled, double-blind clinical trial of hydrogen and oxygen inhalation for treatment of acute exacerbations of chronic obstructive pulmonary disease (AECOPD) was completed in 10 hospitals in China (Table 5-1). The aim of this trial is to investigate whether the inhalation of hydrogen/oxygen mixture was superior to oxygen in improving symptoms. The result demonstrated that hydrogen/oxygen therapy is superior to oxygen therapy in patient with an acute exacerbation of COPD and it has acceptable safety and tolerability profile [Zhong, *et al.*, 2020].

Table 5-1 Hospitals participating in this clinical trial

- The First Affiliated Hospital of Guangzhou Medical University, Guangdong
- The First Hospital of Hebei Medical University, Hebei
- Shanghai Pulmonary Hospital, Shanghai
- Shanghai Fifth People's Hospital, Shanghai
- Tianjin Medical University General Hospital, Tianjin
- Zhongshan Hospital, Fudan University, Shanghai
- Shanghai Tenth People's Hospital, Shanghai
- The First Affiliated Hospital of Zhengzhou University, Henan
- Second Hospital of Shanxi Medical University, Shanxi
- Shanghai East Hospital of Tongji University, Shanghai

Patients and method

Patients, aged 40 years or older, with evidence of clinically acute exacerbation of COPD according to the diagnostic criteria were eligible for this study. All patients had a baseline forced expiratory volume in 1 second (FEV1) less than 80% and FEV1/forced vital capacity (FVC) less than 70% in pulmonary function tests, and had an increase in or new onset of at least two major COPD symptoms (wheezing, sputum production or sputum purulence), or one major COPD symptom plus at least one minor COPD symptom (fever, increased respiratory rate and heart rate [$\geq$ 20% from baseline], cough, wheezing rale and sore throat/rhinorrhea with 5 days) during at least 2 days consecutively and requiring any change of pharmacological intervention. Patients were also required to have a baseline Breathlessness, Cough, and Sputum Scale (BCSS) score of at least 6 points.

All eligible patients were randomly assigned in a 1:1 ratio using a randomisation sequence created by a computer program, to receive either hydrogen/oxygen mixture therapy or oxygen alone therapy. A total of 108 patients were randomly allocated to Hydrogen/oxygen group (n=54) and Oxygen group (n=54).

The hydrogen/oxygen mixture or oxygen were introduced via a nasal mask. The hydrogen/oxygen mixed gas is provided by a new equipment hydrogen/oxygen atomizer (AMS-H-01, Asclepius, Shanghai, China) with a flow rate of 3.0 L/min and a hydrogen/oxygen volume ratio of 67% and 33%. The oxygen for oxygen alone therapy comes from a medical oxygen concentrator with molecular sieve, and the gas flow rate is also 3.0 L/min.

The mean time of gas exposure was 6.4 days (range, 1 to 7 days) for the Hydrogen/oxygen group and 6.4 days (range, 1 to 7 days) for the Oxygen group, with no significant between-group differences.

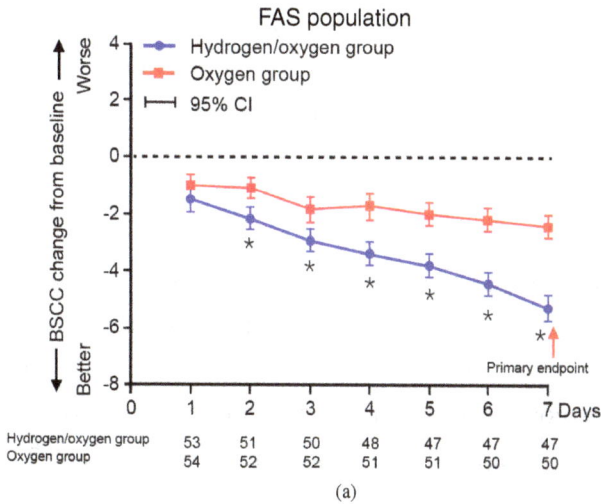

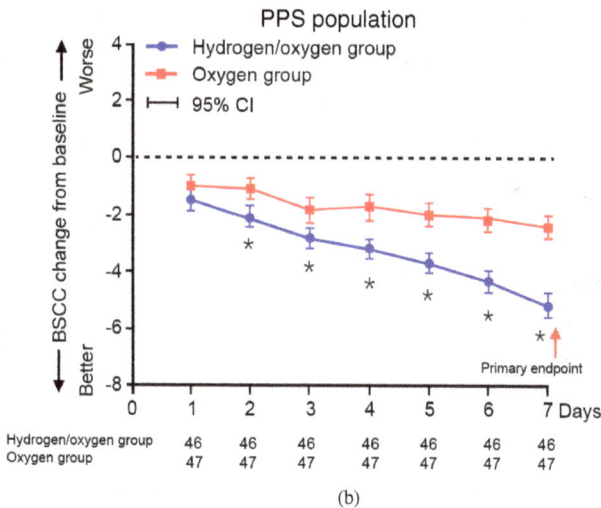

Figure 5-8. Seven-days change from baseline in BCSS score in FAS and PPS population. BCSS, Breathlessness, Cough and Sputum Scale; FAS, full analysis set; PPS, per-protocol set. * p<0.05. Red arrows represent that the BCSS score change from baseline at day 7 is the primary efficacy endpoint.
From Zhong, et al. [2020]

The mean treatment period ranged from 364.9 to 375.4 minutes/day in Hydrogen/oxygen group and 366.0 to 378.5 minutes/day in Oxygen group, without significant between-group differences.

Results

Breathlessness, Cough, and Sputum Scale (BCSS) change: For the primary endpoint in the full analysis set (FAS) opulation, the change from baseline in BCSS score was −5.3 (range, −10 to −1) in the Hydrogen/oxygen group and −2.4 (range, −6 to 0) in Oxygen group (Figure 5-8a). The difference in the primary endpoint was −2.75 (95% CI, −3.27 to −2.22), with the upper confidence limit not more than the superiority limit of 0. Similarly, in the per-protocol set (PPS) population, the change from baseline in BCSS score was −5.2 (range, −8 to −1) in the Hydrogen/oxygen group and −2.69 (range, −6 to 0) in Oxygen group (Figure 3b). The difference in the primary endpoint was −2.69 (95% CI, −3.21 to −2.17), with the upper confidence limit not more than the superiority limit of 0. Improvement from baseline in BCSS score reached significance in patients receiving hydrogen/oxygen therapy compared with controls from day 2 to day 7 (Figure 5-8a and 5-8b).

Cough Assessment Test (CAT) change: With regard to CAT score, there was a statistically significant reduction in the Hydrogen/oxygen group (−11.00 [95% CI, −12.60 to −9.48]) compared to the control (−6.00 [95% CI, −7.46 to −4.61]) in FAS population (p<0.001). The data in PPS population were also consistent with these results (−11.40 [95% CI,

−12.99 to −9.79] vs. −5.90 [95% CI, −7.37 to −4.38], p<0.001). In FAS population, changes from baseline in the pulmonary function parameters did not differ significantly between treatment groups, including FVC (p = 0.309), FEV1 (p = 0.769) and FEV1/FVC (p = 0.536). In addition, the arterial blood gas was measured at day 8 after initial treatment to evaluate the arterial oxygenation. The patients in both treatment groups did not differ in terms of the arterial oxygenation parameters, with no significant differences in pH (p = 0.700), PaO_2 (p = 0.461), $PaCO_2$ (p = 0.160), and HCO^3- (p = 0.136). The consistent results of pulmonary function and arterial oxygenation parameters were observed in the PPS population.

Arterial oxygen saturation (SaO₂) change: The SaO_2 improved more in the Hydrogen/oxygen group compared with the control at day 2 (0.6% vs. −0.5%, p = 0.041) and day 4 (0.7% vs. −0.4%, p = 0.031) in FAS population (Figure 5-9a). Improvement from baseline in SaO_2 reached significance in patients receiving hydrogen/oxygen therapy compared with control at day 4 (0.6% vs. −0.5%, p = 0.041) in PPS population (Figure 5-9b). However, no significant between-group differences were found for the changes in SaO_2 at other time points. No patient received any other oxygen inhalation or noninvasive ventilation during study period, without significant between-group differences.

Adverse events (AEs): Overall, AEs were reported in 34 (63.0%) patients in Hydrogen/oxygen group and 42 (77.8%) patients in Oxygen group, without statistical difference (p = 0.140). All AEs were resolved with

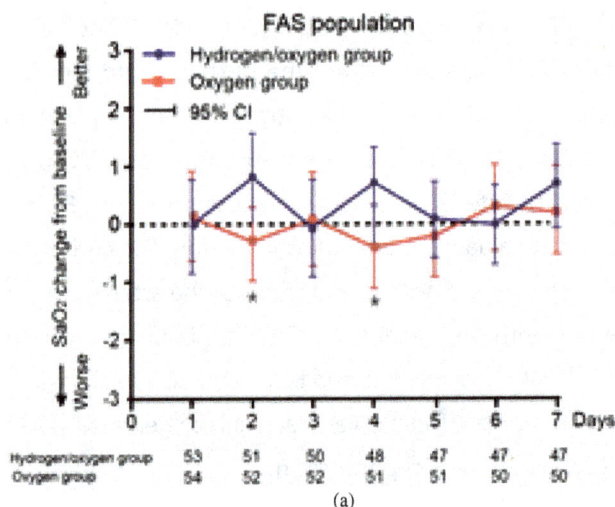

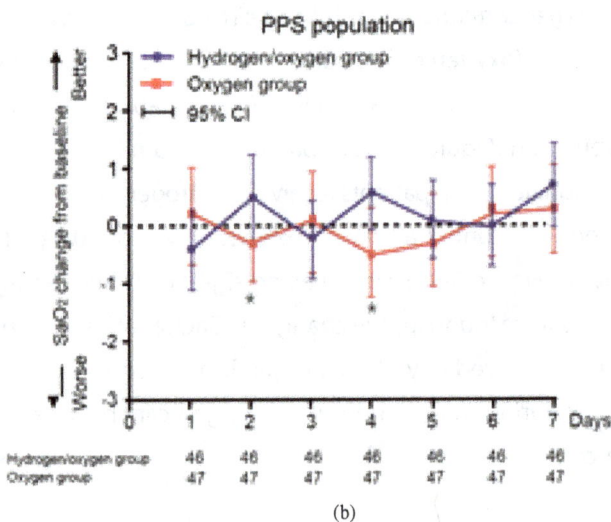

Figure 5-9. Seven-days change from baseline in SaO$_2$ in FAS and PPS population. SaO$_2$, noninvasive arterial oxygen saturation; FAS, full analysis set; PPS, per-protocol set. * $p<0.05$.
From Zhong, *et al.* [2020]

treatment interruption and symptomatic treatment. No notable changes were observed in physical examinations, vital signs, liver and kidney functions. No death and equipment defects were reported during the study period.

Comment

This is the first multicenter, randomized, controlled trial to investigate the efficacy of hydrogen/oxygen mixture in patients with AECOPD. In the clinical treatment of AECOPD, simple oxygen inhalation therapy is widely used, and this group of studies shows that hydrogen/oxygen inhalation therapy has a better effect than oxygen therapy in improving the respiratory function of patients. At the same time, safety analysis shows that this hydrogen-oxygen mixture inhalation therapy is very safe and has acceptable tolerance.

The main goal of AECOPD treatment is to control the patient's key symptoms, such as dyspnea, cough and sputum. The BCSS score is a universal basis for evaluating these symptoms. This study showed that throughout the study period, hydrogen and oxygen inhalation therapy resulted in a more pronounced decrease in BCSS scores than oxygen inhalation alone. CAT, a recognized survey indicator for cough improvement, in the hydrogen-oxygen mixed gas inhalation group, the improvement of the CAT score was significantly better than that in the oxygen-only group. Moreover, the SaO_2 improved more in the Hydrogen/oxygen group compared with the control.

In terms of improving the key symptoms of AECOPD, hydrogen and oxygen inhalation is better than pure oxygen inhalation, mainly due to the anti-inflammatory and antioxidant effects of hydrogen.

The main cause of AECOPD is inflammation. Infection and hypoxia can cause oxidative stress. Inflammation and oxidation can promote each other. Therefore, the application of hydrogen to inhibit inflammation and anti-oxidation is a logical method to treat COPD. Due to its extremely small molecules, hydrogen can carry oxygen molecules on the one hand, and on the other hand can quickly diffuse through the biofilm in the body, so the mixed use of hydrogen and oxygen also further improves hypoxia. The rapid spread of hydrogen molecules throughout the body and cells determines that it can quickly produce curative effects, which undoubtedly has great therapeutic value for AECOPD patients in critical conditions.

This experiment shows that the inhalation of a mixture of hydrogen and oxygen does not produce more adverse reactions than pure oxygen inhalation. In fact, the "adverse events" shown in the trial are not necessarily due to gas inhalation, but may be related to the disease itself and the patient's feelings. Moreover, these adverse events are controllable and tolerable, and disappear soon after interruption of treatment and symptomatic treatment. It is now recognized that hydrogen does not produce special side effects in biology, because normal human intestinal bacteria produce hydrogen, and divers can safely inhale hydrogen for a long time. Because COPD is a common disease, severe cases often require oxygen, and oxygen content of the hydrogen-oxygen mixture used in this experiment is 33%, which is similar to the oxygen content in the clinical oxygen therapy, therefore, there is reason to believe that in the future the simple and inexpensive gas therapy may replace traditional oxygen therapy for long-term use at home.

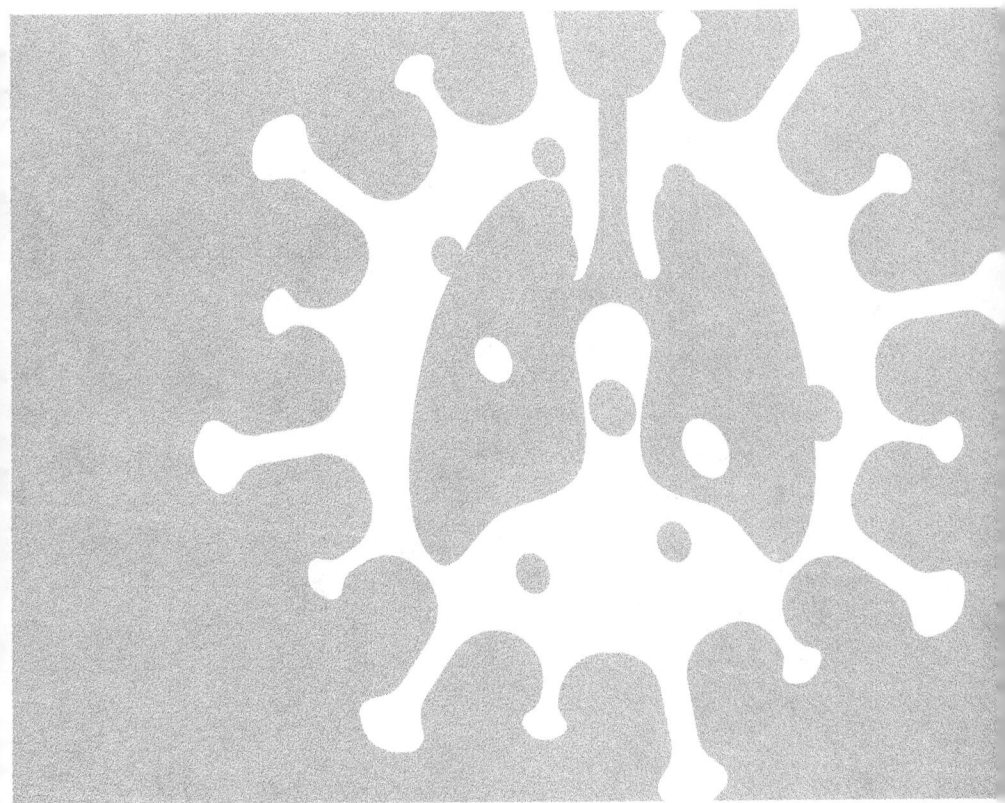

Rationality of Application of Hydrogen-Oxygen Inhalation for COVID-19

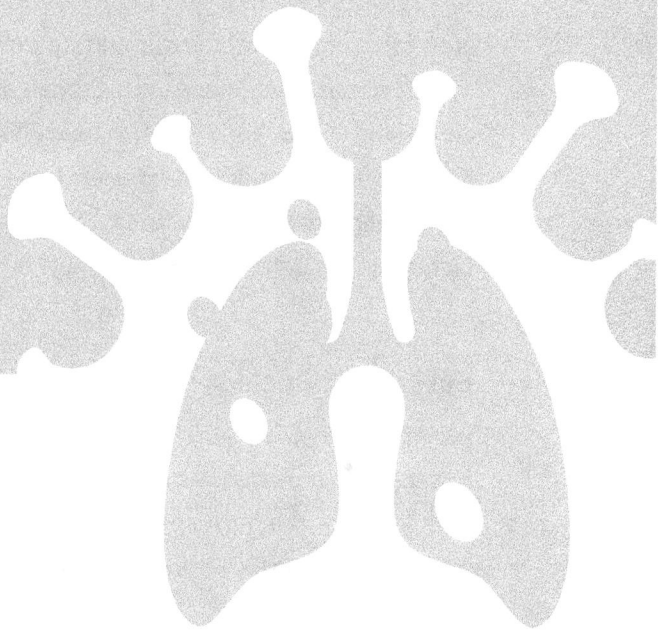

The first 5 chapters introduce the biological role of hydrogen and the study of the effects of hydrogen on experimental lung injury, examine the pathogenesis of lung injury caused by HCoVs including COVID-19, focus on the role of oxidative stress caused by ROS overproduction in the pathogenesis of respiratory viral infections, and review the experimental and clinical studies of hydrogen-oxygen inhalation for treatment of lung diseases. The above-mentioned contents are coherent and complementary. From these descriptions, it can be understood that the use of hydrogen to treat pneumonia and related injury caused by viruses including COVID-19 is theoretically reasonable. Table 6-1 compares the antagonistic effects of hydrogen on various links in the pathogenesis of respiratory viral infections.

COVID-19 is a new type of disease. In the absence of a special antiviral therapy, symptomatic and supportive therapy plays a vital role. China has clinically applied hydrogen-oxygen inhalation therapy containing 66% H_2 and 34% O_2 to treat COVID-19 pneumonia. From the clinical observation and experience, the application of hydrogen-oxygen inhalation therapy for COVID-19 is based on the following facts and considerations (Refer to Table 6-1).

Based on clinical symptoms

Patients with COVID-19 have multiple pulmonary and extra-pulmonary symptoms [Hussin, *et al.*, 2020]. According to reports from Wuhan, China, the most common symptoms at onset of illness are fever (98%), cough (76%), and myalgia or fatigue (44%); less common

Table 6-1 Various links in the pathogenesis of respiratory viruses and the antagonistic effects of hydrogen.

COVID-19 Pathogenesis and Treatment	Biological and Therapeutic Effects of H_2	Reference
ROS overproduction and suppression of antioxidative mechanism, inducing oxidative stress	Scavenging toxic ROS/ RNS and antioxidant effects	Iida, *et al*. [2016]; Huang, *et al*. [2010]; Kawamura, *et al*. [2020]; Ohta [2014]
Abnormal signet expression such as inhibited Nrf2 and HO-1 and up-regulated HMGB1	Down-regulate HMGB1 by activating Nrf2 and HO-1 activity	Khomich, *et al*. [2018]
Cytokine storm and inflammation	Inhibition of pro-inflammatory cytokines and anti-inflammation	Nogueira, *et al*. [2019]; Yao, *et al*. [2019]; Gharib, *et al*. [2001]
Enhanced apoptosis and necrosis	Anti-apoptosis and cytoprotection	Ohta [2014]; Fung and Liu [2019]
Inhibition of autophagy	Increase autophagy	Gassen [2019]
Inhibition of innate and T cell immunity	Increase the activity of NK and T cells	Channappanavar and Perlman [2017]; Xu, *et al*. [2020]
Mitochondrial dysfunction	Maintain mitochondria function	Favreau, *et al*. [2012]; Ishibashi [2019]; Ishihara, *et al*. [2019]
Pro-fibrotic response and fibrosis trend	Down-regulate TGF-β1 activity	Beijing Group of National Research Project for SARS [2003]; Rogel, *et al*. [2011]
Promotion of viral replication through ROS	Scavenging ROS	Khomich, *et al*. [2018]
Obstruction of lower respiratory tract and increased inspiratory effort	Reduce airway resistance and decrease inspiratory effort	Glauser, *et al*. [1969] Zhou, *et al*. [2018]

(Continued)

Table 6-1 (*Continued*)

COVID-19 Pathogenesis and Treatment	Biological and Therapeutic Effects of H_2	Reference
Hyperoxic acute lung injury	Improve hyperoxic lung injury through selectively removing ROS and cytoprotection	Altemeier, *et al.* [2007]; Kawamura, *et al.* [2013]; Audi, *et al.* [2017]
Ventilator-induced lung injury	A protective role against lungs during ventilation through anti-apoptosis and inhibition of inflammation	Huang, *et al.* [2010; 2011]
Damaged epithelial barrier and increased bacterial infection	Maintain epithelial barrier through antioxidation; antisepsis shock	Liu, *et al.* [2013]; Zhang, *et al.* [2016]; Xie, *et al.* [2010]
Aggravated lung injury by complicated hemorrhagic shock and resuscitation (HSR)	Protect the lung parenchyma and improve acute lung injury through anti-inflammation and cytoprotection	Kohama, *et al.* [2015]; Moon, *et al.* [2019]; Meng, *et al.* [2019]

symptoms are sputum production (28%), headache (8%), hemoptysis (5%), and diarrhea (3%). More than half of patients develop dyspnea [Huang, *et al.*, 2020; Lake, 2020].

According to experiences in acute exacerbations of chronic obstructive pulmonary disease (AECOPD) and advanced lung cancer, more than 90% of patients have improved respiratory symptoms after 1–2 weeks of hydrogen-oxygen inhalation, more than 50% of patients have significantly improved, and most patients have significantly improved physical fitness and performance status [Shanghai Asclepius, 2019; Chen, *et al.*, 2019]. Given that for patients with mild and ordinary types of COVID-19, improving symptoms is the first choice for treatment, it is of practical significance to apply hydrogen and oxygen inhalation to eliminate patients' respiratory symptoms and improve physical fitness.

Based on pathological features

Tian, *et al.* [2020] reported two patients with lung adenocarcinoma complicated by COVID-19 infection who underwent lobectomy. Postoperative pathological examination showed that in addition to the tumor, the lungs of both cases show edema, protein exudates, and focal reactive hyperplasia with plaque-like inflammatory cells and multinucleated giant cell infiltration. Since neither patient show symptoms of pneumonia at the time of surgery, these changes represent the early stages of COVID-19. Autopsy results of patients who died of COVID-19 reveal significant alveolar exudative inflammation and interstitial inflammation, alveolar epithelial proliferation, and clear film formation in the lungs. Alveolar infiltrating immune cells are mainly macrophages and monocytes. Most of the infiltrating lymphocytes are CD4-positive T cells. The exudative response is very serious in alveolar tissue, and is more significant than the SARS changes reported in the literature. Small

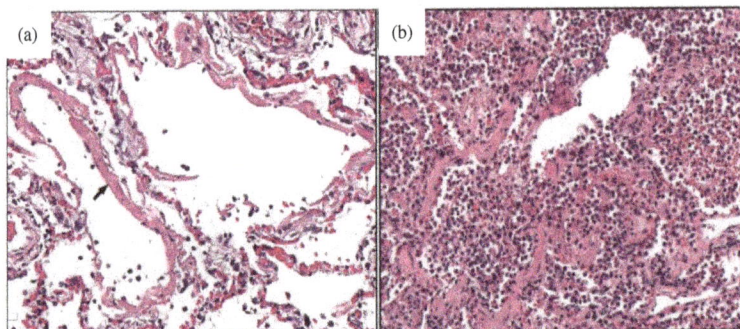

Figure 6-1 (a) Diffuse alveolar damage in the acute stage. Note hyaline membranes (arrow). (b) The airspaces are filled by a mix of neutrophils and histocytes (acute bronchopneumonia).

From Barton, et al. [2020].

airways have a large amount of mucus and high viscosity, which can even obstruct the airways [Yao, *et al.*, 2019; Tang, *et al.*, 2020; Liu, *et al.*, 2020; Barton, *et al.*, 2020].

Clinically, by the end of the first week after COVID-19 infection, the disease can progress to severe pneumonia, respiratory failure, and death in some cases. This progression is associated with extreme rise in inflammatory cytokines, including IL2, IL7, IL10, GCSF, IP10, MCP1, MIP1A, and TNFα [Singhal, 2020].

In view of the fact that COVID-19 is mainly pathologically exudative inflammation and interstitial inflammation of lungs (Figure 6-1) and hydrogen has a significant anti-inflammatory effect [He, *et al.*, 2020; Gong, *et al.*, 2016; Liu, *et al.*, 2018], it is obvious that inhalation of hydrogen-oxygen mixed gas, which is mainly hydrogen, can curb the progress of the disease.

Based on clinical findings

It is clinically found that patients with severe COVID-19 are observed to have increased airway resistance when receiving mechanically assisted breathing, such that although gas is infused at elevated pressure, the patient's blood oxygen saturation does not necessarily improve. Under bronchoscopy, it is often noticed that the distal bronchus accumulates more viscous fluid, inducing airway obstruction (Figure 6-2). It is proved that hydrogen molecules, as the

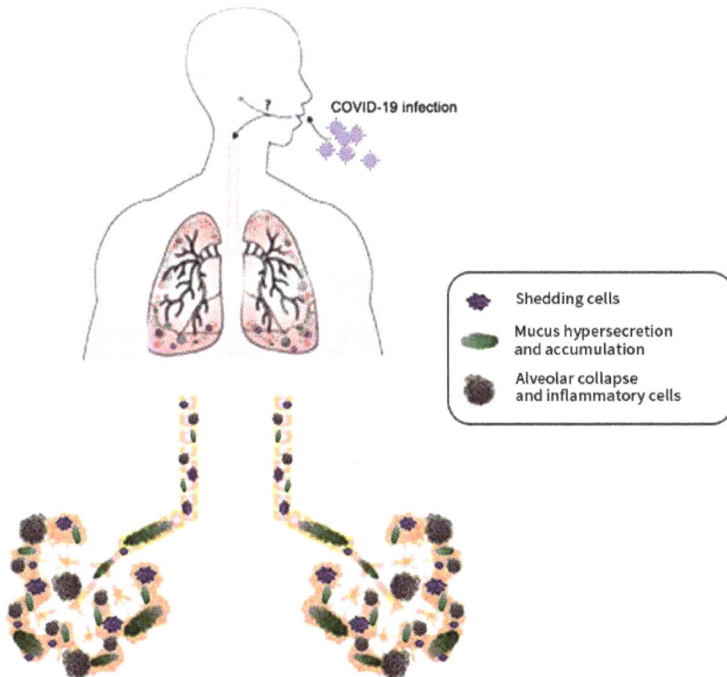

Figure 6-2 The proposed model for distal airway obstruction in COVID.

smallest in size, can carry oxygen into the distant bronchi, improving hypoxia.

Based on adverse effects of hyperoxic and mechanical ventilation

As mentioned in Chapter 2, high oxygen intake and the use of a ventilator for mechanical positive pressure assisted breathing can induce inflammation and lung toxicity, called hyperoxic acute lung injury (HALI) and ventilator-induced lung injury (VILI), and even promote the occurrence of respiratory failure. Hydrogen has the effect of inhibiting inflammation and cytoprotection, which can prevent and improve the unfortunate acute lung injury caused by these treatment procedures.

Based on multiple organ lesions

Among patients with COVID-19 reported in Wuhan, China, 11% have multiple organ failure [Chen, et al., 2020]. Huang, et al. [2020] reported that acute fulminant myocarditis is found in 12% of patients with COVID-19. Xu, et al. [2020] examined the autopsy pathology of a patient with COVID-19 who had ARDS and found that the liver and heart show typical ARDS-like histological changes similar to those of the lung, with lymphocyte infiltration as the main feature, and liver tissue showing moderate microvascular steatosis.

Clinically, some patients with COVID-19 show neurologic signs, such as headache, nausea, and vomiting. Increasing evidence shows that the coronaviruses are not always confined to the respiratory tract and that they may also invade the central nervous system inducing neurological injury. The infection of SARS-CoV has been detected in the brains from both patients and experimental animals, where the brainstem is heavily infected. Furthermore, some coronaviruses have been demonstrated to be able to spread via a synapse-connected route to the medullary cardiorespiratory center from the mechanoreceptors and chemoreceptors in the lung and lower respiratory airways [Li, et al., 2020]. In situ hybridization confirms the presence of HCoV RNA in brain parenchyma outside blood vessels.

Clinical investigation also shows that abnormal liver function test results have been observed in patients with COVID-19, making the liver the most frequently damaged organ outside of the respiratory system [Li and Fan, 2020]. Increasing evidence has highlighted the close relationship of abnormal liver biochemistries with severity of COVID-19. In the cohort of 1099 patients with COVID-19 from China, about 30% have increased activity of transaminase, which is significant in severe and critical cases.

Severe or critical patients have laboratory characteristic findings of septic shock and multiple organ dysfunction or failure, such as liver injury, renal injury, and heart injury.

Hydrogen has been recognized as a "philosophical molecule" [Hirano, et al., 2020]. Due to its small molecule and strong penetrating power, hydrogen can quickly pass through the biofilm and reach a high concentration in the cell, thereby exerting a wide range of biological effects. The beneficial effects of hydrogen is documented in more than 170 disease models and human diseases [Tao, *et al.*, 2019] ,including heart [Li, *et al.*, 2020; Zhao, *et al.*, 2019], vascular [Guan, *et al.*, 2019], brain [Li, *et al.*, 2018], renal [Guan, *et al.*, 2019; Guan, *et al.*, 2019], liver [Fukuda, *et al.*, 2007], and hematologic diseases [Qian, *et al.*, 2019]. Therefore, it is reasonable to believe that in the case of COVID-19, inhalation of hydrogen-oxygen will help improve the state of the whole body and maintain the functions of various organs.

Based on the safety of hydrogen

Hydrogen is a physiological gas [Levitt, 1980], and normal human intestinal bacteria produce hydrogen all the time [Strocchi, *et al.*, 1994]. According to Levitt's report [1969], the average daily hydrogen production of bacteria in the intestinal tract of normal people is 345.6 mL; after eating, the amount of H_2 produced increases 7–30 times. Calculated at 7 times, the H_2 production is 292.18 L/day, and at 30 times, it can reach up to 1252.8 L/day. At present, the "Hydrogen-Oxygen Atomizer" used in clinical practice has a maximum gas flow rate of 3 L/min and contains 67% hydrogen gas. The actual gas entering the lung is estimated to be 20% of the inhaled volume. According to this calculation, the hydrogen inhalation per day is 47.52–95.4 L, which is far lower than the amount of hydrogen produced in the body after eating under physiological conditions [Levitt, 1980; Strocchi, *et al.*, 1994]. Hydrogen has long been used as a useful gas for commercial diving to relieve high-pressure neurological syndrome [Levitt, 1969]. Therefore, clinically, hydrogen-oxygen inhalation can be applied for a long time without worrying about its side effects.

Based on the simplicity of the therapy

The convenience of any clinical treatment is very important, especially for severe patients. The hydrogen-oxygen inhalation system uses a nasal catheter or mask inhalation method (Figure 6-3), which can be used alone or together with conventional oxygen inhalation and mechanically assisted breathing. Since the inhaled hydrogen-oxygen mixed gas contains 34% oxygen, it is actually equivalent to simultaneous oxygen inhalation. In view of the simplicity of the method of use, the hydrogen-oxygen inhalation therapy can be used in rehabilitation centers or at home for patients in the rehabilitation period.

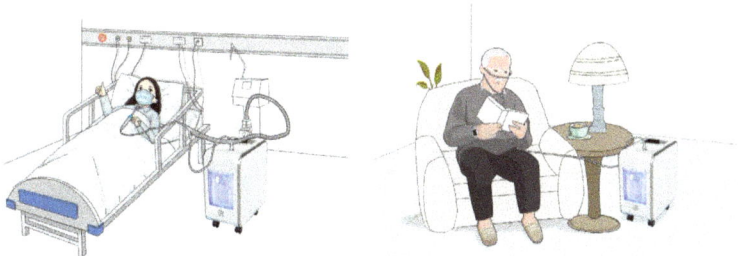

Figure 6-3   The hydrogen-oxygen inhalation therapy can be used in hospital or at home.

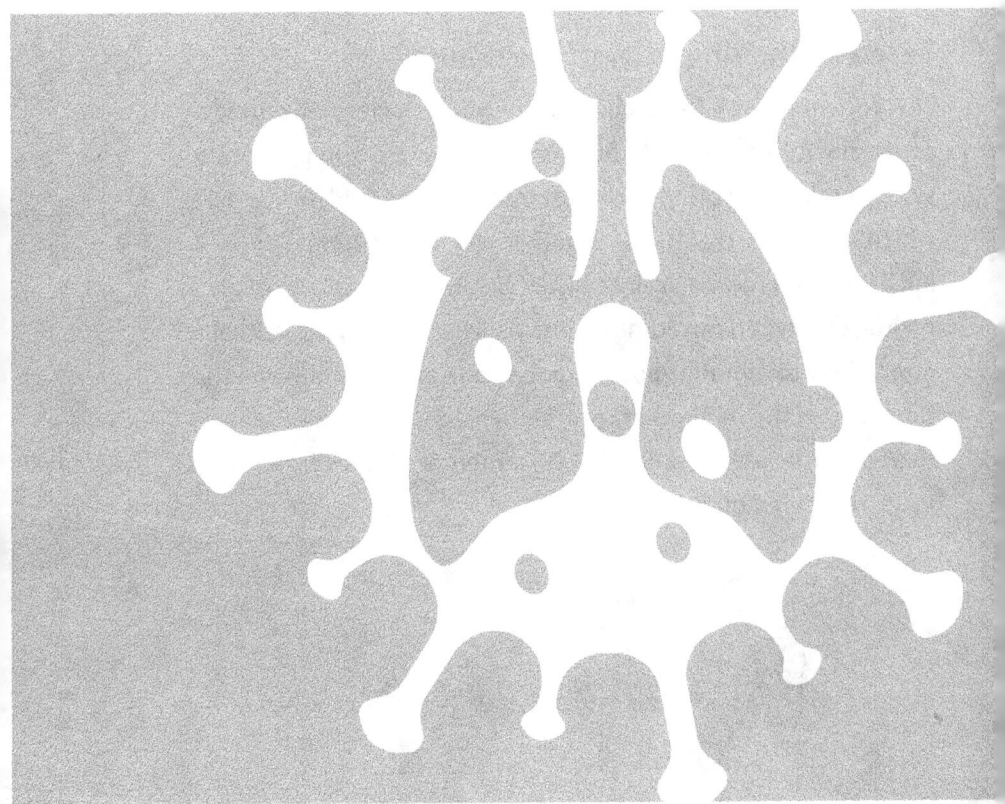

Clinical Use of Hydrogen-Oxygen Inhalation for Treatment of COVID-19

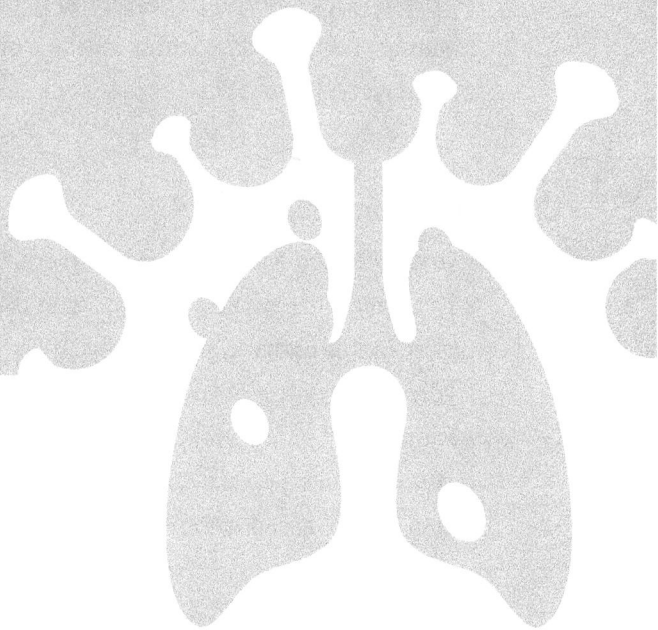

Real World Evidence survey of treatment for 259 patients with COVID-19

From February 3 to March 19, 2020, 259 patients with COVID-19 who voluntarily received hydrogen-oxygen inhalation were investigated by a *real world evidence* (RWE) survey in 18 hospitals in China.

Patients

All patients were hospitalized and diagnosed with COVID-19 after nucleic acid testing, chest CT, and clinical examination based on China's *COVID-19 Diagnosis and Treatment Plan (Trial Version 7)*.

The number of patients undergoing the RWE survey in each hospital was a maximum of 43, a minimum of 2 and a median of 10 (Table 7-1). The length of hospital stay before hydrogen-oxygen treatment was 0–44 days, with an average of 17.19 days and a median of 17 days (Figure 7-1).

Treatment method

Without changing the original treatment, the patient continuously or intermittently inhaled the hydrogen-oxygen mixture through a nasal cannula or mask, and the inhalation flow was 3 L/min, using a Hydrogen-Oxygen Atomizer (AMS-H-01, provided by Shanghai Asclepius, SFDA registration number 20203080066), in which the mixed gas consisting of 67% H_2 and 33% O_2 was produced from pure water. Before receiving the hydrogen-oxygen inhalation treatment,

Table 7-1 Hospitals and number of cases participating in the RWE survey.

Hospital	Cases	%
Guangzhou 8th People Hospital, Guangdong	43	16.6
Jinzhou People Hospital, Hubei	36	13.90
Leishenshan Hospital, Hubei	30	11.58
Shenzhen 3rd People Hospital, Guangdong	24	9.27
Wuhan Hankou Hospital, Hubei	23	8.88
1st Affiliated Hospital of Nanchang University, Jiangxi	18	6.95
Sheshou Hospital of Traditional Chinese Medicine, Hubei	15	5.79
Wuhan Hanyang Hospital, Hubei	15	5.79
Harbin 6th People Hospital, Heilongjiang	12	4.63
Jiangling People Hospital, Hubei	10	3.86
Jingzhou City Central Hospital, Hubei	9	3.47
Songzi City People Hospital, Hubei	9	3.47
Suihua Cancer Hospital, Hubei	4	1.54
Hubei Integrated Chinese and Western Medicine Hospital, Hubei	3	1.16
Gongan Hospital of Traditional Chinese Medicine, Hubei	2	0.77
Jianli Hospital of Traditional Chinese Medicine, Hubei	2	0.77
Qiqihaer City 1st Hospital, Heilongjiang	2	0.77
Wuxue City 1st People Hospital, Hubei	2	0.77
Total	**259**	**100**

the patients carefully listened to the doctor's introduction to the performance, efficacy, and adverse reactions of the AMS-H-01 machine, and signed the "informed consent" forms. The method and time of inhaling hydrogen-oxygen were completely determined by the patients.

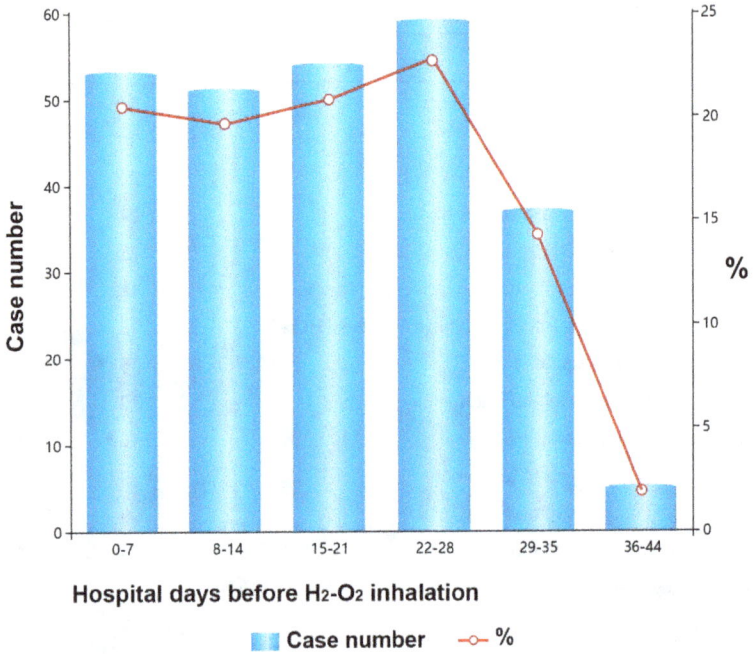

Figure 7-1 The length of hospital stay (days) before hydrogen-oxygen treatment in 259 patients with COVID-19.

Evaluation

The patients were evaluated for the severity of the disease and related symptoms at two time points: "the first treatment" (referring to the treatment with inhaled hydrogen-oxygen) and "the last treatment" (after the last hydrogen-oxygen inhalation). The severity of the disease was graded 0 to 3, in order of mild, moderate, severe, and very severe. The relevant symptoms that were evaluated include fever, cough, expectorant, shortness of breath, chest tightness, chest pain, and dyspnea. Except for fever, other symptoms were graded on a scale of 0 to 4, with none, mild, moderate, severe, and very severe. The patient's peripheral blood oxygen saturation (SpO_2) was evaluated.

Results

Time of hydrogen-oxygen inhalation

The treatment period of 259 patients receiving hydrogen-oxygen inhalation was 2–28 days, with an average of 7.05 days and a median of 7 days. The cumulative treatment time of 222 cases was 0.2–324 hours, with an average of 80.24 hours and a median of 56 hours (Figure 7-2).

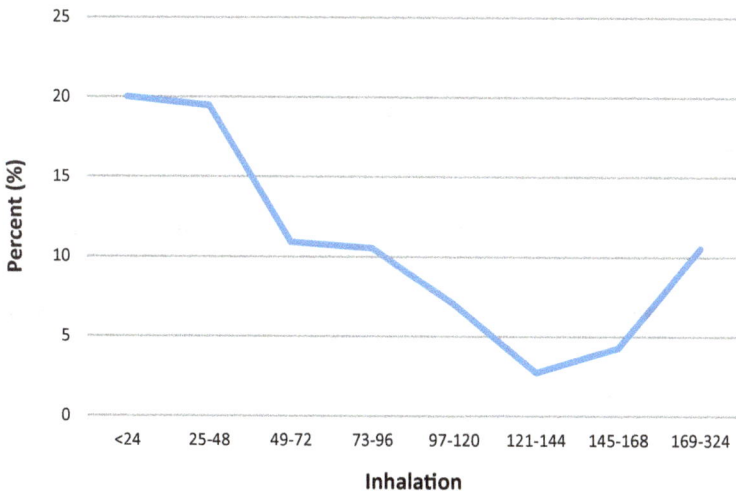

Figure 7-2 The cumulative time (hours) of hydrogen-oxygen gas inhalation in 222 patients with COVID-19.

Improvement of symptoms

In 259 patients with COVID-19, almost all symptoms and peripheral blood oxygen saturation improved, and the severity of the disease decreased after receiving hydrogen-oxygen inhalation for one week. Statistical analysis showed that all the above indexes were significantly different after 7 days of hydrogen-oxygen inhalation compared with before the treatment (Table 7-2).

Table 7-2 259 cases of COVID-19 patients before and after treatment with hydrogen-oxygen inhalation.

| Variables | Case | Grading* | Rating at Follow-up Points Median/Mean | | P Value* |
			First[x]	Last[x]	
Disease severity	240	0–3, M,Mo,S,vS	2.000/1.603	2.000/2.050	2.096e-13**
Fever	253	Fever, no fever	9.09%	1.19%	5.104e-05**
Cough	252	0–4, N,M,Mo,S,vS	0.000/0.702	0.000/0.246	<2.2e-16**
Expectorant	252	0–4, N,M,Mo,S,vS	0.000/0.349	0.000/0.095	7.33e-09**
Shortness of breath	251	0–4, N,M,Mo,S,vS	0.000/0.653	0.000/0.255	9.654e-12**
Chest tightness	250	0–4, N,M,Mo,S,vS	0.000/0.592	0.000/0.224	4.329e-11**
Chest pain	251	0–4, N,M,Mo,S,vS	0.000/0.0383	0.000/0.2440	3.413e-06**
Dyspnea	248	0–4, N,M,Mo,S,vS	0.000/0.440	0.000/0.153	2,886e-08**
SpO_2	199		96%	97%	7.517e-15**

*The severity of the disease is divided into M (mild), Mo (moderate), S (severe), and vS (very severe); symptoms are classified as N (none), M (mild), Mo (moderate), S (severe), and vS (very severe).

[x]"First" means before receiving hydrogen-oxygen treatment and "Last" means after receiving hydrogen-oxygen treatment.

** p < 0.001; ≠Analysis: McNemar test for fever, Wilcoxon rank sum test for other variables.

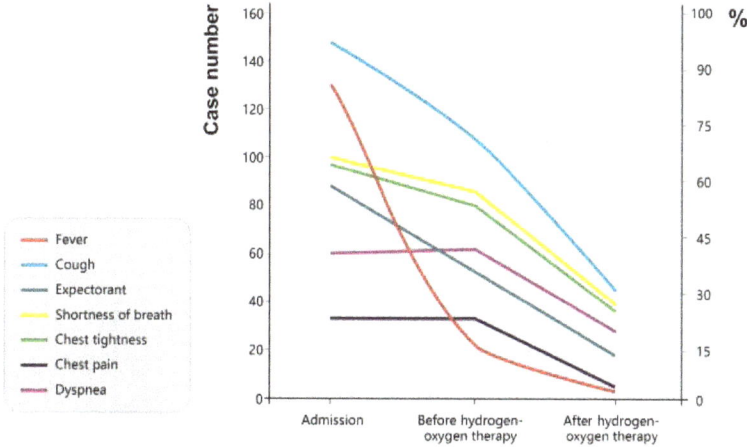

Figure 7-3 Changes in various individual symptoms after hydrogen-oxygen inhalation.

The changes in various individual symptoms after hydrogen-oxygen inhalation are shown in Figure 7-3. All symptoms, including fever, cough, expectorant, shortness of breath, chest tightness, chest pain, and dyspnea had significantly improved. Those who had fever at first had their body temperature lowered to normal. The most significant improvement was seen in patient's dyspnea. When starting hydrogen-oxygen therapy, the number of patients with dyspnea was almost the same as that at the time of admission, and after 7 days of hydrogen-oxygen therapy, all patients' dyspnea improved or disappeared.

A total of 199 patients underwent follow-up for peripheral blood oxygen saturation (SpO$_2$), showing a significant improvement after H$_2$-O$_2$ inhalation compared with before (Figure 7-4) (p = 7.517, e-15 < 0.001).

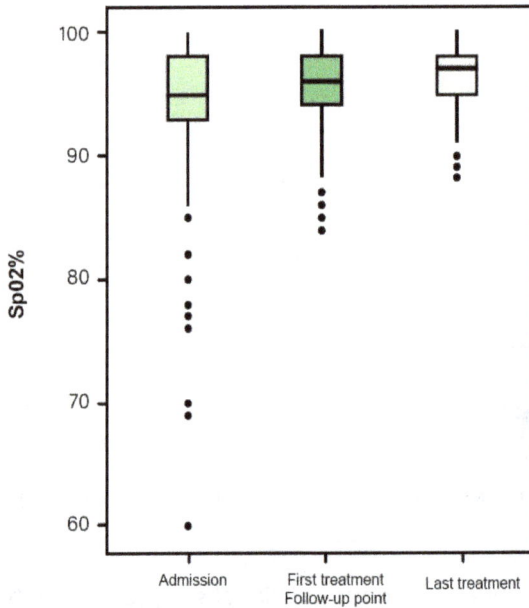

Figure 7-4 SpO$_2$ change before and after H$_2$-O$_2$ inhalation.

Hydrogen and oxygen inhalation for adjuvant treatment of COVID-19 patients: *Real World* research report

This study screened a total of 103 COVID-19 patients who were hospitalized in 11 wards of medical care from January 2020 to March 2020 (Table 7-3) [Guan, *et al.*, 2020]. The patients were divided into study groups and control groups according to whether inhalation of mixed hydrogen and oxygen gas were used for adjuvant therapy (exposure factors). The groups were 52 cases and 51 cases respectively. In the study group, 8 patients who had no dyspnea

Table 7-3 Hospitals and researchers participating the trial

	Hospitals	Researchers
1	Leishenshan Hospital (Wuhan, Hubei) and Guangdong Province Hospital of Traditional Chinese Medicine (Guangdong)	Xu Zou
2	Guangzhou 8th People Hospital (Guangdong)	Liang Leichun
3	Hankou Hospital of Wuhan City (Hubei) and The 1st Affiliated Hospital of Guangzhou Medical University (Guangdong)	Chen Ailian
4	Wuxue 1st People Hospital (Hubei)	Yang Jianming
5	Hanyang Hospital of Wuhan (Hubei) and Weifang Weien Hospital (Shandong)	Wei Chunhua
6	Haerbin 6th Hospital (Heilongjiang)	Li Xiaodong
7	Suihua Cancer Hospital (Hubei)	Zhu Wenyu
8	Jingzhou Central Hospital (Hubei)	Hu qinming
9	Shishou Hospital of Traditional Chinese Medicine (Hubei)	Sun Xiaochong
10	Wuhan Cancer Hospital (Hubei)	Guo Guangyun
11	Shanghai 5th People Hospital (Shanghai) and Leishenshan Hospital (Hubei)	Shi Jindong

before admission were excluded. A total of 44 patients were finally included for the analysis. In the control group, 3 patients who had no dyspnea at the time of admission and 2 patients who had no dyspnea before admission were excluded. A total of 46 patients were finally included for the analysis.

There were no significant differences in the average age, gender distribution, disease severity, peripheral blood oxygen saturation (SpO_2), fever degree, and cough level between the two groups of subjects at the time of entry (P>0.05). The symptoms of dyspnea, shortness of breath, chest tightness and chest pain in the study group were slightly heavier than those in the control group (P<0.05).

However, the following indicators are different between the two groups: the number of days of hospitalization before admission was 16.2±8.3 days in the study group, 3.8±4.1 days in the control group (P<0.001), and the number of days of treatment after admission was 7.8±3.4 days in the study group , the control group was 10.8±3.9 days (P<0.001), the total number of days of treatment (to the last treatment day) was 24.1±8.4 days in the study group, and 14.6±3.8 days in the control group (P<0.001).

All subjects in the study group inhaled hydrogen and oxygen mixed gas through a nasal catheter using a novel device, Hydrogen/ Oxygen Atomizer (AMS-H-01, Shanghai, China), at flow rate of 3.0 L/min and hydrogen/oxygen volume ratio of 67%: 33%. The median cumulative inhalation time of hydrogen and oxygen in the study group was 64.0 (24.0–157.0) hours, and the median daily treatment time was 7.7 (6.0–18.3) hours. The control group did not receive hydrogen and oxygen gas treatment.

The results are shown below.

Clinical improvement rate

The main efficacy indicator of this study is the clinical improvement rate after the last treatment. Clinical improvement is defined as a decrease in the severity of the disease by at least one level. The clinical improvement rate refers to the ratio of the number of patients whose disease degree has improved to the total number of cases. The results of this study showed that compared with the day of first therapy, the clinical improvement rate was 20.5% and 2.3% (P=0.019), respectively,

Table 7-4 Comparison of improvement rate between the study group and control group

Time	Group	Cases	Improvement rate (%)	P value	RR	95% CI
2nd day after therapy	Study	44	20.5	—	—	—
	Control	44	2.3	0.019	9	(1.2, 68.1)
3rd day after therapy	Study	44	31.8	—	—	—
	Control	44	11.4	0.038	2.8	(1.1, 7.1)
After last therapy	Study	44	70.5	—	—	—
	Control	44	31.8	<0.001	2.2	(1.4, 3.6)

Note 1: Two subjects in the control group failed to obtain the disease severity rating after the last therapy and were treated as missing values.

Note 2: RR: relative risk; 95% CI: 95% confidence interval. The comparison of count data between groups was tested by chi-square test/fisher exact probability method.

on the second day of treatment, and 31.8% and 11.4%(P=0.038), respectively, on the third day of treatment in the study group and in the control group. Compared with the baseline, the clinical improvement rate after the last therapy in the study group reached 70.5%, and the control group reached 31.8%. The difference was statistically significant (P<0.001) (Table 7-4).

Dyspnea improvement rate

The improvement of dyspnea is defined as a decrease in the symptom grade by at least 1 grade (the symptom grade is divided into 0 to 4, indicating no, mild, moderate, severe, and extremely severe). The improvement rate refers to the proportion of the number of patients whose symptoms have improved to the total number of cases.

Compared with the day of the first therapy, the improvement rate of dyspnea was 50% and 23.9%, respectively, in the study group and in the control group on the second day of treatment. The difference between the two groups was statistically significant (P=0.019). However, on the third day of treatment and after the last treatment, the difference of improvement rate of dyspnea in both groups was not statistically significant (Table 7-5). This fact suggests that within 24 hours (the next day) after the inhalation of hydrogen and oxygen, the dyspnea is improved quickly.

When analyzing the rating of dyspnea severity based on continuous data, the dyspnea level of the study group from baseline (from the first day) showed improvement, no matter on the second day of treatment (P<0.05) or the third day (P = 0.001) and after the last treatment (P=0.001), the improvement rating was all higher than that of the control group, and the difference in mean improvement between the two groups was statistically significant (Table 7-6).

Table 7-5 The comparison of dyspnea improvement rate between two groups

Time	Groups	Cases	Dyspnea improvement rate(%)	P value	RR	95%CI
2nd day after therapy	Study	44	50.0	—	—	—
	Control	46	23.9	0.019	2.1	(1.2, 3.8)
3rd day after therapy	Study	44	70.5	—	—	—
	Control	46	56.5	0.249	1.2	(0.9, 1.7)
After last therapy	Study	44	93.1	—	—	—
	Control	46	91.3	>0.999	1.0	(0.9, 1.2)

RR: relative risk; 95% CI: 95% confidence interval. The comparison of count data between groups was tested by chi-square test/fisher exact probability method.

Table 7-6 Improvement rating of the dyspnea in two groups

Time	Group	Cases	Improvement rating of the dyspnea	P value	Mean difference	95%CI
2nd day after therapy	Study	44	0.7 (0.9)	—	—	—
	Control	46	0.2 (0.4)	0.003	0.5	(0.2, 0.8)
3rd day after therapy	Study	44	1.1 (1.0)	—	—	—
	Control	46	0.5 (0.5)	0.001	0.6	(0.2, 1.0)
After last therapy	Study	44	1.9 (1.0)	—	—	—
	Control	46	1.2 (0.8)	0.001	0.7	(0.3, 1.1)

Improvement rating = score on the second day of treatment (/day 3/last day)-score on the day of first treatment, expressed as a mean (standard deviation); Mean difference: difference between the mean; 95% CI: 95% confidence interval. Two independent samples t test was used to compare continuous measurement data between groups.

The patients with dyspnea was further divided into two subgroups according to the severity of the disease at the time of enrollment, which was mild, common, severe, and critical. Compared to the baseline (the day of the first treatment), the improvement ratings of the dyspnea of the two subgroups, on the second, third day and after the last treatment were seen in Table 7-7, the difference between the study and the control group was >0 points, and the difference in the mean improvement was all statistical significance (P<0.05).

The common symptoms of COVID-19, such as shortness of breath, chest tightness, chest pain, and cough, were significantly improved after inhalation of hydrogen and oxygen. The improvement rate of various symptoms is seen in Table 7-8.

If the symptom rating was analyzed according to continuous data, the improvement rating of the symptoms in the study group was significant compared with the baseline (the day of the first

Table 7-7 Improvement rating of the dyspnea in patients with subgroups of different severity

Subgroups of severity	Time	Groups	Cases	Improvement rating	P value	Mean difference	95%CI
Mild and common	2nd day after therapy	Study	22	0.7 (1.0)	—	—	—
		Control	15	0.1 (0.4)	0.024	0.6	(0.1, 1.0)
	3rd day after therapy	Study	22	1.0 (1.0)	—	—	—
		Control	15	0.3 (0.6)	0.014	0.7	(0.2, 1.3)
	After end therapy	Study	22	1.7 (0.9)	—	—	—
		Control	15	1.1 (0.5)	0.024	0.6	(0.1, 1.0)
Severe and critical	2nd day after therapy	Study	22	0.7 (0.8)	—	—	—
		Control	29	0.3 (0.5)	0.028	0.4	(0.1, 0.9)
	3rd day after therapy	Study	22	1.2 (1.0)	—	—	—
		Control	29	0.7 (0.5)	0.021	0.5	(0.1, 1.0)
	After end therapy	Study	22	2.1 (1.0)	—	—	—
		Control	29	1.2 (1.0)	0.005	0.9	(0.3, 1.4)

Improvement rating = score on the second day of treatment (/day 3/last day)-score on the day of the first treatment, expressed as a mean (standard deviation); Mean difference: difference between means; 95% CI: 95% confidence interval. Two independent samples t test was used to compare continuous measurement data between groups.

treatment). The results showed that for common symptoms of COVID-19 such as shortness of breath, chest tightness, chest pain and cough, the difference of the mean is >0 points compared with the control group, and the difference of the improvement mean is statistically significant (Table 7-9).

Peripheral blood oxygen saturation (SpO$_2$)

The improvement of the SpO$_2$ value in the resting state of the study group from the baseline (the day of the first treatment) was seen on

Table 7-8 The improvement rate of various symptoms after hydrogen-oxygen inhalation

Symptoms	2nd day of the therapy		3rd day of the therapy		Day after last therapy	
	Study (%)	Control (%)	Study (%)	Control (%)	Study (%)	Control (%)
Shortness of breath	63.6	23.9*	72.7	58.7	90.7	82.6
Chest tightness	51.2	23.9*	76.7	47.8**	81.4	63.0
Chest pain	40.9	0.0*	45.2	2.2*	54.6	6.5*
Cough	45.5	13.0**	59.1	30.4**	79.6	60.9

* $P<0.001$, ** $P<0.05$

Table 7-9 Improvement rating of symptoms from baseline after hydrogen-oxygen inhalation

Symptoms	2nd day of the therapy		3rd day of the therapy		Day after last therapy	
	Study	Control	Study group	Control	Study	Control
Shortness of breath	1.0 (0.9)	0.2 (0.5)*	1.3 (0.1)	0.6 (0.6)*	2.0 (1.0)	1.1 (0.8)*
Chest tightness	0.8 (0.9)	0.2 (0.6)*	1.2 (1.0)	0.4 (0.8)*	1.7 (1.2)	1.0 (1.1)*
Chest pain	(0.5 (0.8)	0.0 (0.1)*	0.7 (0.9)	0.0 (0.1)*	0.9 (0.1)	0.1 (0/2)*
Cough	0.5 (0.7)	0.1 (0.4)*	1.0 (1.0)	0.3 (0.5)**	1.6 (1.1)	0.8 (0/8)*

Improvement rating = score on the second day of treatment (/day 3/last day)-score on the day of first treatment, expressed as a mean (standard deviation); Mean difference: difference between the mean; 95% CI: 95% confidence interval. Two independent samples t test was used to compare continuous measurement data between groups. * $P<0.001$, **$P<0.05$.

the second day of treatment (95% CI = 0.4–1.8, P<0.05) and the third day (95% CI = 0.9–2.7 P<0.001) and after the last treatment (95% CI = 0.9–3.3, P=0.001), the mean value of the difference compared with the control group was >1%, and the difference in the improvement mean was statistically significant. In the study group, 24 subjects had hydrogen and oxygen inhalation time shorter than (or equal to) the overall median. However, it was still found that the SpO_2 of these patients improved from the baseline (the day of the first treatment), and after the last treatment, the difference in the mean between the study group and the control group was greater than 1% also, and the difference in average improvement was statistically significant ($P<0.05$).

Adverse events

Adverse events mainly refer to whether laboratory tests (blood routine, liver function, kidney function, and blood biochemistry), disease severity, and clinical symptoms (dyspnea, shortness of breath, chest tightness, chest pain, and cough) have worsened during the study. The occurrence of adverse events: 6 cases (10 case-times) of adverse events occurred in the study group, and 13 cases (31 case-times) occurred in the control group. The incidence of adverse events was 13.6% and 28.3%, respectively. There was no difference between the two groups ($P>0.05$).

Comment

This is a retrospective cohort analysis that investigates the *real world* of COVID-19 patients after receiving hydrogen and oxygen mixture inhalation treatment. The results are encouraging. Almost all patients' symptoms such as dyspnea, shortness of breath, chest tightness, chest pain, and coughing improved significantly on the second and third days after inhaling a mixture of hydrogen and oxygen. These improvements were maintained after the last treatment was completed. At the same time, the severity of the disease has improved accordingly. SpO_2 also showed an increase. This effect is particularly significant if the improvement rating was analyzed according to continuous data. Statistical analysis showed that, regardless of the symptom improvement rate or the daily improvement rating, the difference was always significant compared with the control group that did not receive hydrogen and oxygen inhalation therapy.

A retrospective cohort controlled study on the effect of hydrogen and oxygen inhalation on the length of hospital stay in COVID-19 patients

This study is a retrospective cohort *real world* survey based on medical records, targeting COVID-19 patients who were hospitalized from January 2020 to March 2020 in 3 treatment centers of Wuhan Leishenshan Hospital and Jiangling County People's Hospital in Hubei Province, China. The purpose of the research is to investigate whether the inhalation of mixed hydrogen and oxygen as an adjuvant therapy is beneficial to reduce the days of hospital stay. All study subjects were diagnosed as common type of COVID-19 based on *China's COVID-19 Diagnosis and Treatment Plan (Trial version 7)*.

Subjects and Methods

A total of 180 patients were used as selection subjects for research and they all received conventional treatment. Of these cases, 42 received hydrogen-oxygen inhalation as adjuvant therapy, and the remaining 138 received no such treatment. The hydrogen and oxygen adjuvant therapy adopted the inhalation method (using Hydrogen and Oxygen Atomizer AMS-H-01, Asclepius, Shanghai,

China), inhaling a mixed gas containing 67% H_2 and 33% O_2 through a nasal cannula or a face mask, and the gas flow rate was 3000 ml/min. Inhalation time exceeded 6 hours per day.

According to the selection and exclusion criteria, cohort controlled study subject was determined. The age, gender, location of the patient's hospitalization, and the number of days from disease onset to hospitalization were used as independent variables, the propensity score matching (PS) method was used to match the treatment group and the control group according to whether or not the patient received auxiliary hydrogen and oxygen therapy. From 42 patients who received hydrogen and oxygen inhalation adjuvant therapy and 138 patients who did not receive such treatment, respectively, 32 cases in each of the hydrogen and oxygen group and the control group were matched. The log rank test was used to compare the difference in the length of hospital stay between the two groups.

Results

The result is shown in Figure 7-5. The average length of stay in the hydrogen and oxygen group was 5 days shorter than that in the control group, and the median length of stay was 1.5 days shorter. The difference between the groups was statistically significant (p = 0.0081).

Comment

COVID-19 is still raging around the world. A large number of patients put great pressure on families, medical institutions and the whole

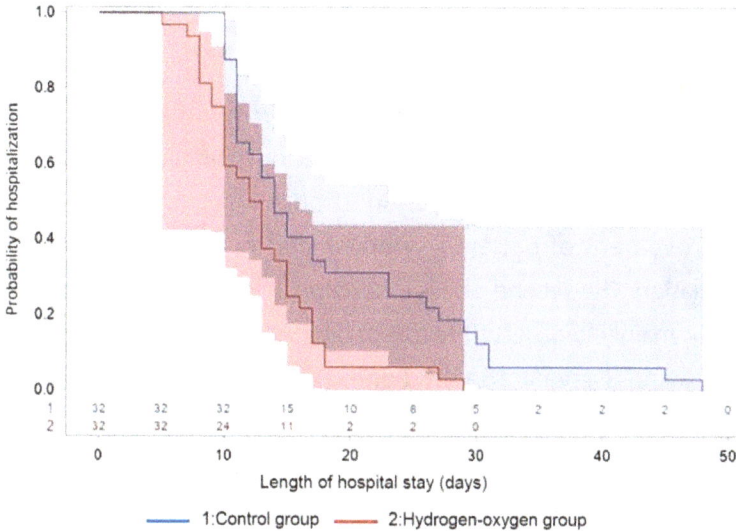

Figure 7-5 The Length of hospitalization in hydrogen and oxygen inhalation group and control group.

Note: The research was led by Zhong Nanshan, Guan Weijie and Shi Jindong. This is a pre-report of the research results, and the detailed results will be published in the official paper later.

society. The shortening of the patient's hospital stay is of great significance to both the patient and the society. This retrospective *real world* survey now shows that patients who receive hydrogen and oxygen inhalation as adjuvant therapy have an average hospital stay of 5 days shorter than those of the control group who did not receive the adjuvant therapy. The median length of hospital stay was reduced by 1.5 days. The results show that the inhalation of hydrogen and oxygen mixture, as an adjuvant treatment for COVID-19 patients, is beneficial to reduce the stay days in the hospital.

Discussion and illustrated cases

Among the above three clinical studies, the first one is a multi-center "*real world evidence*" survey. Patients under investigation receive hydrogen-oxygen inhalation therapy without changing the original treatment. The "self-control" method is used to observe the improvement of patients' symptoms after hydrogen-oxygen inhalation. The second one is a retrospective multi-central cohort study, mainly to observe the role of hydrogen-oxygen inhalation in improving dyspnea. The third one is to investigate whether the inhalation of mixed hydrogen and oxygen as an adjuvant therapy is beneficial to reduce the days of hospital stay. The results of these studies are basically similar and they are as follows:

(1) Hydrogen-oxygen inhalation can quickly improve the patient's breathing difficulties. Generally, the shortness of breath improves after 24 hours of inhalation. Patients' symptoms of laborious breathing exercise, open mouth breathing, inflamed nose, and sitting breathing improved accordingly;

(2) Cough, chest tightness, and chest pain are the most common symptoms of COVID-19 pneumonia patients. All symptoms continue to improve rapidly after inhalation of hydrogen and oxygen;

(3) SpO_2 also increases successively after hydrogen and oxygen inhalation;

(4)   In terms of the severity of the disease, all patients showed improvement, and none of them worsened during or after the treatment.

(5)   Hydrogen and oxygen inhalation adjuvant therapy can shorten the patient's hospital stay, which is of great significance to patients, medical institutions and society.

Hydrogen-oxygen inhalation is very safe. Among a total of more than 300 patients enrolled in the three studies, no major adverse reactions are reported. Aiming at the risk of explosion and combustion of high-concentration hydrogen, the AMS- H-03 Hydrogen-Oxygen Atomizer has a special design and device, including the so-called zero-gas cavity storage, pipeline multi-layer flame arrest, hydrogen concentration detection, etc., which successfully eliminates the above-mentioned risks and the safety of the facility is guaranteed (Chinese safety certificate CMTC QW2019 No. 414 and patent CN105624724B and CN103789784B).

COVID-19 is a new disease. This extremely infectious disease is unfamiliar to medical staff, patients, and society. Although the overall mortality rate is not high, the concentration of many deaths in the short term will undoubtedly cause great psychological panic in patients, their relatives, and society, including uninfected healthy people. Therefore, adopting a simple method without special side effects to quickly improve patients' symptoms not only reduces patients' pain and promotes recovery, but also has great significance for reducing the social fear of this disease and stabilizing the mental state of the person.

At COVID-19 treatment centers, many patients appear very excited and grateful as their symptoms improve after receiving hydrogen-oxygen inhalation therapy. On-site medical staff have recorded many videos of moving scenes. Some typical cases are featured as follows.

Case 1

Female, 63 years old. In early February 2020, there was no obvious cause of dry cough, which gradually worsened, accompanied by wheezing and fatigue. February 2, chest CT examination revealed multiple patchy lesions in both lungs. SpO_2 was below 85%. COVID-19 nucleic acid test was positive. Diagnosed as COVID-19. High-flow oxygen inhalation and symptomatic treatment were given. After 2 weeks, the patient's cough improved and the nucleic acid test turned negative. In the case of mask oxygen supply, the patient's SpO_2 could be maintained at more than 90%, but could not be separated from oxygen inhalation. Breathing was still short, complaining of chest tightness. She started receiving hydrogen-oxygen inhalation on February 28, 8 hours a day. After 2 days, the patient's shortness of breath and chest tightness disappeared. One week later, the patient could get out of bed and move freely without oxygen inhalation; SpO_2 remained above 95%; CT review showed that most of the lung lesions were absorbed (Figure 7-6).

Case 2

Female, 57 years old. On January 29, 2020, the patient developed fever, cough, and dyspnea, and she received antibiotics, oxygen

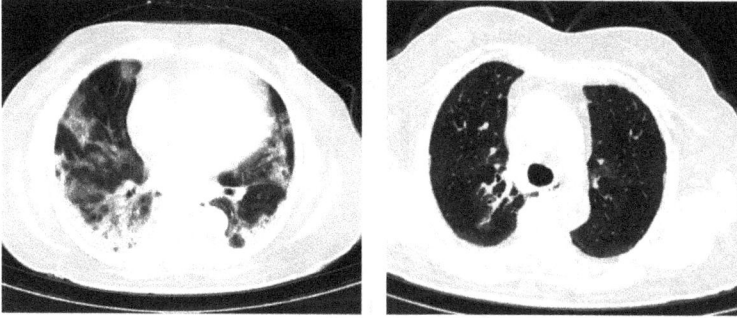

Figure 7-6 Left: Chest CT before hydrogen-oxygen inhalation show multiple patchy lesions in both lungs. Right: Chest CT after 14 days of hydrogen-oxygen inhalation show that most of the pulmonary lesions were absorbed.

inhalation, and other symptomatic treatments. Her condition progressed, body temperature rose to 40°C, SpO_2 decreased to 70%, consciousness was blurred, and stool and urinary incontinence developed. Chest CT showed "large white shadows" on both lungs. Given a ventilator to assist breathing. Half a month later, her body temperature dropped to normal range and her cough improved, but she felt persistent chest tightness and chest pain. In the case of high flow oxygen inhalation, SpO_2 could reach 95%, but it quickly decreased to below 90% after stopping oxygen inhalation. A CT scan of the chest on February 16 showed a large number of residual lesions. At 10 am on February 22, the patient began to inhale hydrogen-oxygen. After an hour, the patient felt "especially comfortable". Three days later, the patient got rid of the oxygen treatment and ventured to the corridor outside her ward freely. Together with several "hydrogen friends" who also received hydrogen-oxygen inhalation, she invited the medical staff to take a photo and share their happiness (Figure 7-7). On February 27, chest

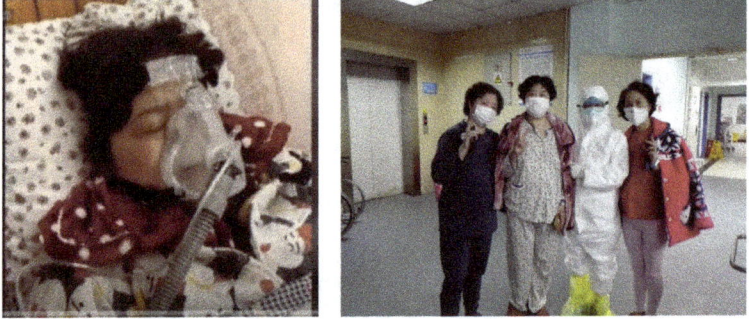

Figure 7-7 Left: The patient inhaling mixed hydrogen-oxygen gas. Right: The patient and her "hydrogen friends", benefiting from hydrogen-oxygen treatment, invite doctors to take photos and share their healthy happiness together.

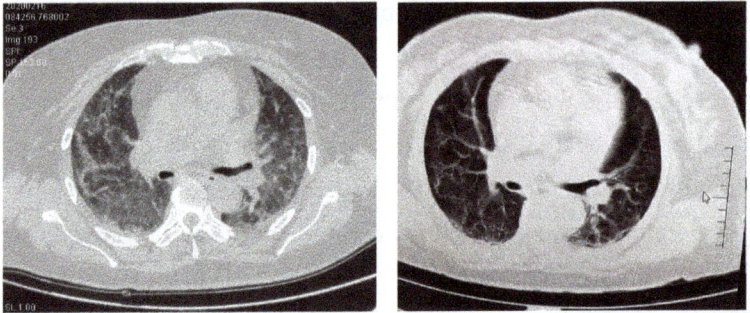

Figure 7-8 Left: CT before hydrogen-oxygen inhalation show multiple inflammatory lesions in lungs. Right: CT images taken 5 days after inhalation of hydrogen-oxygen show significant absorption of inflammation in both lungs.

CT was reviewed, and inflammation in the lungs was basically absorbed (Figure 7-8). On February 29, when Dr. Zhong Nanshan was invited to discuss COVID-19 treatment with colleagues from the European Society of Respiratory Disease, the patient excitedly expressed her feelings for the hydrogen-oxygen inhalation therapy. She said: "I'm so happy! How many days have I been ill? I have never been as comfortable as I am now. The Hydrogen-Oxygen Atomizer is so amazing, I am very grateful."

Case 3

Male, 37 years old. On January 27, 2020, he was admitted to the hospital due to fever, coughing, dyspnea, and wheezing for one week. Chest CT showed diffuse shadows in both lungs and COVID-19 RNA was positive in pharyngeal swabs. SpO_2 was reduced to a minimum of 80%. Diagnosed as COVID-19 (severe type), acute respiratory failure. Given high-flow oxygen inhalation through the mask and the nasal canal, as well as intravenous infusion of gamma globulin, albumin, and corticosteroids. After 2 weeks, the body temperature gradually returned to normal range, the cough was decreased, and the lung CT showed an improvement of acute exudative lesions, but the patient still had significant shortness of breath after mild activity. Without oxygen inhalation, SpO_2 dropped to about 85%, accompanied by chest tightness and chest pain. From March 11, the patient stopped regular oxygen inhalation and changed to inhalation treatment of hydrogen-oxygen mixed gas (67% hydrogen, 33% oxygen) at a flow rate of 6 L/min, inhaling more than 6 hours a day. The patient's shortness of breath improved after 3 days, and chest pain and tightness disappeared after a week. SpO_2 maintained above 97% without oxygen inhalation. Follow-up CT showed absorption of most inflammation in both lungs (Figure 7-9). Multiple consecutive viral RNA tests showed negative results. On March 16, 2020, the patient was discharged from the hospital.

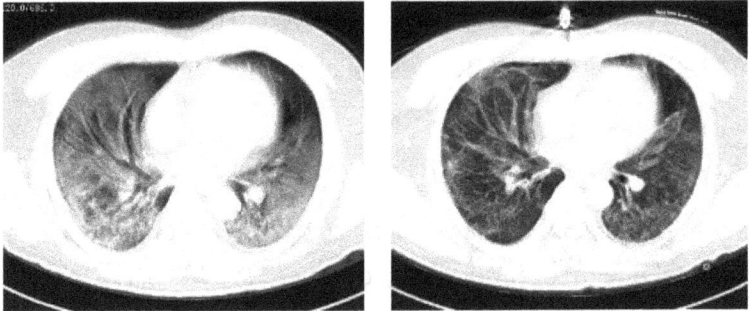

Figure 7-9 Left: CT before hydrogen-oxygen inhalation show diffuse inflammation lesions. Right: CT taken 2 weeks after hydrogen-oxygen inhalation show significant improvement of inflammation of lungs.

During the follow-up period of one month, the patient felt normal.

Case 4

Female, 46 years old. She was admitted to the hospital on February 18, 2020 due to high fever, cough, wheezing, and dyspnea. Temperature 40.1ºC, breathing 40/min, heart rate 140/min, systolic blood pressure 80 mmHg, and SpO$_2$ 82%. Chest CT showed extensive inflammatory exudative lesions in both lungs. Pharyngeal swab COVID-19 nucleic acid test was positive. The diagnosis of COVID-19 (very severe type) was confirmed. The patient was sent to the ICU and received high-flow oxygen inhalation. Dyspnea did not improve. The patient was given tracheal intubation and ventilator-assisted breathing until March 2, when the ventilator was removed, and later on, the tracheal intubation was removed. The nucleic acid test turned negative. SpO_2 increased to 96%. Chest CT showed that most of the lung inflammation disappeared. However, the patient still has intractable cough, shortness of breath, chest pain, and chest tightness. She was in low mood and in a state of depression throughout the day. Symptomatic treatment had no obvious response. From March 18, the patient underwent inhalation of hydrogen-oxygen mixed gas (H_2 67%, O_2 33%) for 6 hours a day. After 2 days, the above symptoms began to improve, and almost completely disappeared after 2 weeks. The change of score of symptoms after hydrogen-oxygen inhalation was followed-up based on Self Reporting Inventory (ACL 90) as in Figure 7-10.

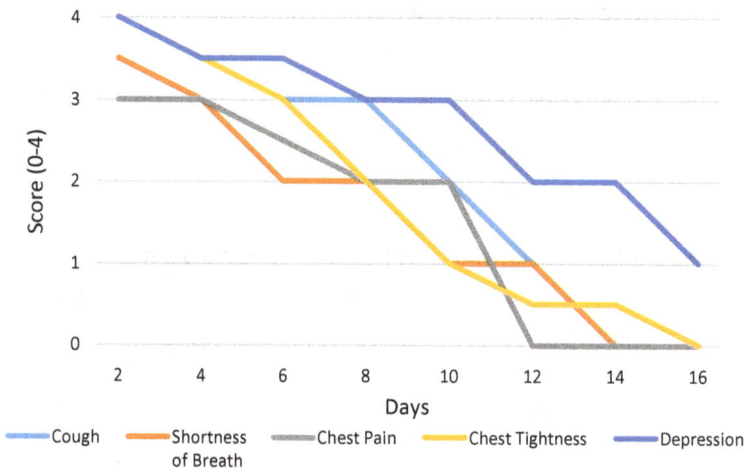

Figure 7-10 The score of symptoms after hydrogen-oxygen inhalation based on Self Reporting Inventory (ACL 90).

Conclusion and recommendations

Although COVID-19 is a self-limiting disease, it is extremely contagious. With the global pandemic, there will be more and more deaths. Clinical observations in China have shown that the early symptoms of the disease can be lacking or mild, but after a period of time, the condition can worsen dramatically. Once severe, the mortality rate reaches 60%. Hydrogen has a wide range of biological effects. Therefore, in the comprehensive treatment of COVID-19, it is reasonable and feasible to offer the hydrogen-oxygen inhalation therapy.

According to existing research and experience, the clinical application of hydrogen-oxygen treatment must follow the following principles:

- Hydrogen and oxygen mixed gas should be inhaled, not pure hydrogen. Inhaling 33% of O_2 is physiologically desirable. Hydrogen can bring oxygen deep into the airways, improving oxygen supply. Inhalation of pure hydrogen will "squeeze out" oxygen and cause hypoxia;

- High concentration of hydrogen should be inhaled, and it is hoped that hydrogen will fill the entire body in a short time. The currently set hydrogen concentration is 67%;

- The inhaled gas should have a sufficient flow rate. When treating severe patients with airway resistance, the flow rate must not be less than 3000 ml/min;

- The inhalation time should be long enough and not less than 2 hours/day; in severe cases, it should be more than 6 hours/day;

- Nasal catheter or mask can be used for inhalation. Patients should be trained to ensure that normal breathing is consistent with "inhaled hydrogen".

In view of the uncertainty of COVID-19, as well as the simplicity and cheapness of this treatment method, hydrogen-oxygen inhalation is recommended for most or all patients, and it is particularly recommended for the following cases:

- For ordinary patients. The purpose of conventional hydrogen-oxygen inhalation is to improve symptoms, especially dyspnea, and to prevent progression to severe illness;

- For critically ill patients. In comprehensive treatment, especially in cases receiving hyperoxia inhalation and mechanical ventilation, hydrogen-oxygen inhalation can improve the efficacy and relieve hyperoxia- or mechanical ventilation-induced lung injury while ensuring sufficient oxygen intake;

- For patients in recovery. Hydrogen-oxygen inhalation can eliminate residual symptoms and is expected to prevent or reduce pulmonary fibrosis and possible sequelae. Using this treatment at home is recommended.

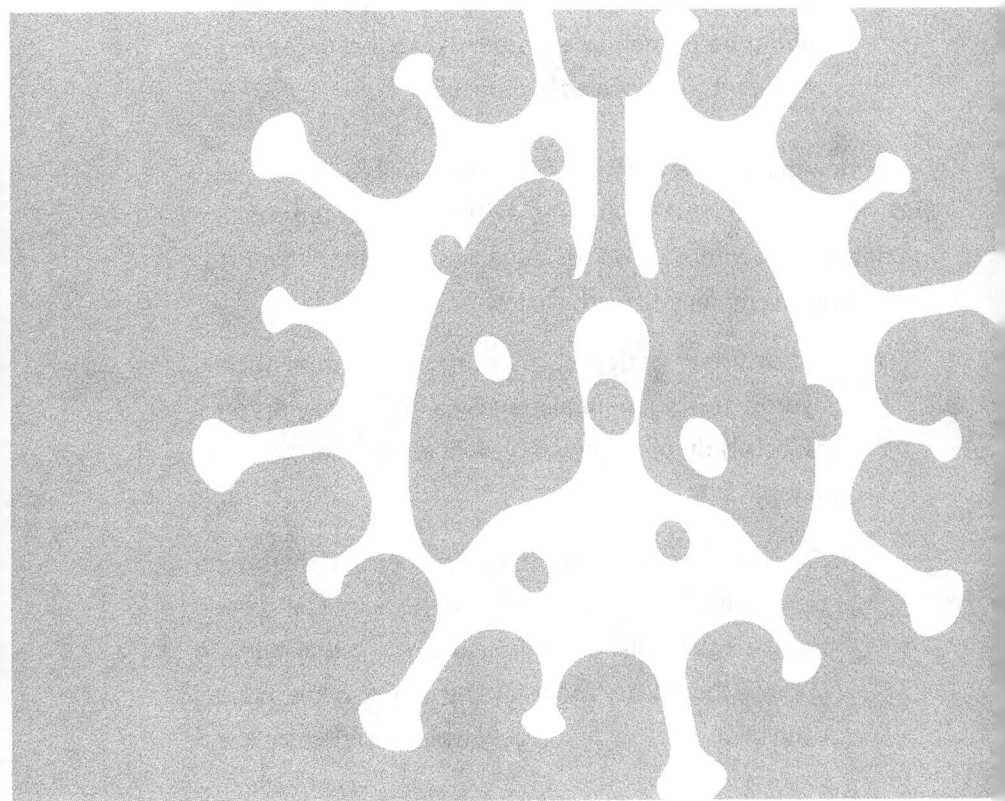

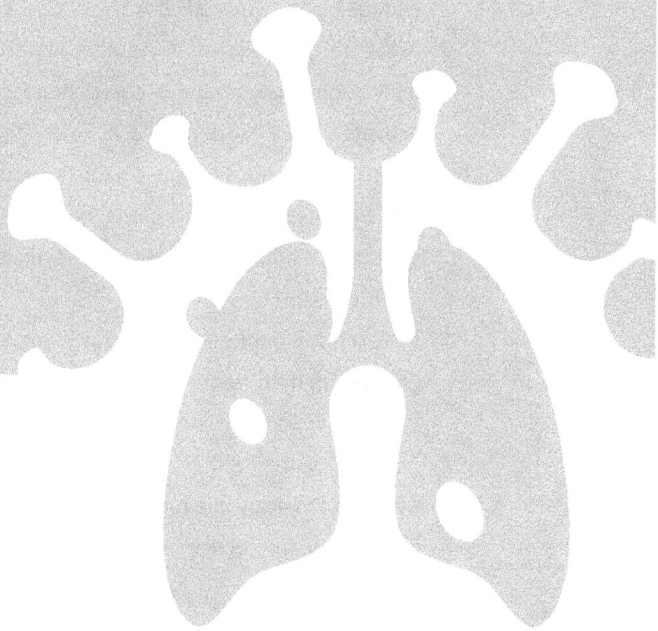

References

1. Akagi J, Baba H. (2019). Hydrogen gas restores exhausted CD8+ T cells in patients with advanced colorectal cancer to improve prognosis. *Oncol Rep.* 41(1), pp. 301–311.

2. Akaike T, Nishida M, Fujii S. (2013). Regulation of redox signalling by an electrophilic cyclic nucleotide. *J Biochem.* 153(2), pp. 131–138.

3. Akira M, Suganuma N. (2014). Acute and subacute chemical-induced lung injuries: HRCT findings. *Eur J Radiol.* 83(8), pp. 1461–1469.

4. Al-Jamal R, Ludwig MS. (2001). Changes in proteoglycans and lung tissue mechanics during excessive mechanical ventilation in rats. *Am J Physiol Lung Cell Mol Physiol.* 281, pp. L1078–1087.

5. Altemeier WA, Sinclair SE. (2007). Hyperoxia in the intensive care unit: Why more is not always better. *Curr Opin Crit Care.* 13(1), pp. 73–78.

6. Altenhöfer S, Radermacher KA, Kleikers PW, *et al.* (2015). Evolution of NADPH oxidase inhibitors: selectivity and mechanisms for target engagement. *Antioxid Redox Signal.* 23(5), pp. 406–427.

7. Amatore D, Sgarbanti R, Aquilano K, *et al.* (2015). Influenza virus replication in lung epithelial cells depends on redox-sensitive pathways activated by NOX4-derived ROS. *Cell Microbiol.* 17(1), pp. 131–145.

8. Angus D, Yang L, Kong L, *et al.* (2007). Circulating high-mobility group box 1 (HMGB1) concentrations are elevated in both uncomplicated pneumonia and pneumonia with severe sepsis. *Crit Care Med.* 35(4), pp. 1061–1067.

9. Aubert RD, Kamphorst AO, Sarkar S, Vezys V. (2011). Antigen-specific CD4 T -cell help rescues exhausted CD8 T cells during chronic viral infection. *Proc Natl Acad Sci USA.* 108, pp. 21182–21187.

10. Audi SH, Jacobs ER, Zhang X, *et al.* (2017). Protection by inhaled hydrogen therapy in a rat model of acute lung injury can be tracked in vivo using molecular imaging. *Shock.* 48(4), pp. 467–476.

11. Bao X, Sinha M, Liu T, *et al*. (2008). Identification of human metapneumovirus-induced gene networks in airway epithelial cells by microarray analysis. *Virology*. 374(1), pp. 114–127.

12. Barton LM, Duval EJ, Stroberg E, Ghosh S, Mukhopadhyay S. (2020). COVID-19 autopsies, Oklahoma, USA. *Am J Clin Pathol*. pii: aqaa062.

13. Beijing Group of National Research Project for SARS. (2003). Dynamic changes in blood cytokine levels as clinical indicators in severe acute respiratory syndrome. *Chin Med J (Engl)*. 116, pp. 1283–1287.

14. Belding ME, Klebanoff SJ, Ray CG. (1970). Peroxidase-mediated virucidal systems. *Science*.167(3915), pp. 195–196.

15. Bhandari V, Rayman Choo-Wing R, *et al*. (2006). Hyperoxia causes angiopoietin 2–mediated acute lung injury and necrotic cell death. *Nat Med*. 12(11), pp. 1286–1293.

16. Bo L, Li C, Chen M, *et al*. (2018). Application of electrocautery needle knife combined with balloon dilatation versus balloon dilatation in the treatment of tracheal fibrotic scar stenosis. *Respiration*. 95, pp. 182–187.

17. Brigham KL. (1986) Role of free radicals and lung injury. *Chest*. 89(6), pp. 859–863.

18. Brydon EW, Morris SJ, Sweet C. (2005). Role of apoptosis and cytokines in influenza virus morbidity. *FEMS Microbiol Rev*. 29(4), pp. 837–850.

19. Buchholz BM, Kaczorowski DJ, Sugimoto R, *et al*. (2008). Hydrogen inhalation ameliorates oxidative stress in transplantation induced intestinal graft injury. *Am J Transplant*. 8(10), pp. 2015–2024.

20. Bulua AC, Simon A, Maddipati R, *et al*. (2011). Mitochondrial reactive oxygen species promote production of proinflammatory cytokines and are elevated in TNFR1-associated periodic syndrome (TRAPS). *J Exp Med*. 208(3), pp. 519–533.

21. Bysani GK, Kennedy TP, Ky N, *et al.* (1990). Role of cytochrome P-450 in reperfusion injury of the rabbit lung. *J Clin Invest.* 86, pp. 1434–1441

22. Casola A, Garofalo RP, Haeberle H, *et al.* (2001). Multiple cis regulatory elements control RANTES promoter activity in alveolar epithelial cells infected with respiratory syncytial virus. *J Virol.* 75(14), pp. 6428–6439.

23. Chalmers S, Khawaja A, Wieruszewski PM, *et al.* (2019). Diagnosis and treatment of acute pulmonary inflammation in critically ill patients: The role of inflammatory biomarkers. *World J Crit Care Med.* 8(5), pp. 59–71.

24. Channappanavar R and Perlman S. (2017). Pathogenic human coronavirus infections: Causes and consequences of cytokine storm and immunopathology. *Semin Immunopathol.* 39(5), pp. 529–539.

25. Channappanavar R and Perlman S. (2020). Evaluation of activation and inflammatory activity of myeloid cells during pathogenic human coronavirus infection. *Methods Mol Biol.* 2099, pp. 195–204.

26. Channappanavar R, *et al.* (2016). Dysregulated type I interferon and inflammatory monocyte-macrophage responses cause lethal pneumonia in SARS-CoV-infected mice. *Cell Host Microbe.* 19(2), pp. 181–193.

27. Chapman KE, Sinclair SE, Zhuang D, *et al.* (2005). Cyclic mechanical strain increases reactive oxygen species production in pulmonary epithelial cells. *Am J Physiol Lung Cell Mol Physiol.* 289, pp. L834–841.

28. Chen C , Zhang XR , Ju ZY, He WF. (2020). [Advances in the research of mechanism and related immunotherapy on the cytokine storm induced by coronavirus disease 2019]. *Zhonghua Shao Shang Za Zhi.* 36(6), pp. 471–475. [in Chinese].

29. Chen J, Qi T, Liu L, *et al.* (2020). Clinical progression of patients with COVID-19 in Shanghai, China. *J Infect.* pii: S0163-4453(20) 30119-5.

30. Chen JB, Kong XF, Xu KC, *et al.* (2019). "Real world survey" of hydrogen-controlled cancer: A follow-up report of 82 advanced cancer patients. *Med Gas Res.* 9(3), pp. 115–121.

31. Chen JB, Qian W, Xu KC, *et al.* (2020). Hydrogen reverse of immune senescence in NSCLC patients. *Med Gas Res.* (in press)

32. Chen N, Zhou M, Dong X, *et al.* (2020). Epidemiological and clinical characteristics of 99 cases of 2019 novel coronavirus pneumonia in Wuhan, China: A descriptive study. *Lancet.* 395(10223), pp. 507–513.

33. Chen X, Wang K, Xing Y, *et al.* (2014). Coronavirus membrane-associated papain-like proteases induce autophagy through interacting with Beclin1 to negatively regulate antiviral innate immunity. *Protein Cell.* 5, pp. 912–927.

34. Cho HY, Jedlicka AE, Reddy SP, *et al.* (2002). Linkage analysis of susceptibility to hyperoxia. Nrf2 is a candidate gene. *Am J Respir Cell Mol Biol.* 26, pp. 42–51

35. Choi G, Wolthuis EK, Bresser P, *et al.* (2006). Mechanical ventilation with lower tidal volumes and positive end-expiratory pressure prevents alveolar coagulation in patients without lung injury. *Anesthesiology.* 105, pp. 689–695.

36. Chu H, Zhou J, Wong BH-Y, *et al.* (2016). Middle East respiratory syndrome coronavirus efficiently infects human primary T lymphocytes and activates the extrinsic and intrinsic apoptosis pathways. *J Infect Dis.* 213(6), pp. 904–914.

37. Circu ML. and Aw TY. (2010). Reactive oxygen species, cellular redox systems, and apoptosis. *Free Radic Biol Med.* 48, pp. 749–762.

38. Comstock AT, Ganesan S, Chattoraj A, *et al.* (2011). Rhinovirus-induced barrier dysfunction in polarized airway epithelial cells is mediated by NADPH oxidase 1. *J Virol.* 85(13), pp. 6795–6808.

39. COVID-19 Infectious Pneumonia Diagnosis and Treatment Plan (Trial Version 7). China National Health Committee and the State Administration of Traditional Chinese Medicine.2020.

40. Crawford A, Angelosanto JM, Kao C, *et al.* (2014). Molecular and transcriptional basis of CD4+ T cell dysfunction during chronic infection. *Immunity.* 40(2), pp. 289–302.

41. Daiber A, Steven S, Weber A, *et al.* (2017). Targeting vascular (endothelial) dysfunction. *Br J Pharmacol.* 174(12), pp. 1591–1619.

42. Damiani E, Adrario E, Girardis M, *et al.* (2014). Arterial hyperoxia and mortality in critically ill patients: A systematic review and meta-analysis. *Crit Care.* 18, pp. 711.

43. Diao M, Zhang S, Wu L, *et al.* (2016). Hydrogen gas inhalation attenuates seawater instillation-induced acute lung injury via the Nrf2 pathway in rabbits. *Inflammation.* 39(6), pp. 2029–2039.

44. Dias-Freitas F, Metelo-Coimbra C, *et al.* (2016). Molecular mechanism underlying hyperoxia acute lung injury. *Respir Med.* 119, pp. 23–28

45. Dikalov S. (2011). Cross talk between mitochondria and NADPH oxidases. *Free Radic Biol Med.* 51(7), pp. 1289–1301.

46. Dole M, Wilson FR, Fife WP. (1975). Hyperbaric hydrogen therapy: a possible treatment for cancer. *Science.* 190(4210), pp. 152–154.

47. Dolinay T, Kim YS, Howrylak J, *et al.* (2012). Inflammasome-regulated cytokines are critical mediators of acute lung injury. *Am J Respir Crit Care Med.* 185, pp. 1225–1234.

48. Dong A, Yu Y, Wang Y, *et al.* (2018). Protective effects of hydrogen gas against sepsis-induced acute lung injury via regulation of mitochondrial function and dynamics. *Int Immunopharmacol.* 65, pp. 366–372.

49. Dos Santos CC and Slutsky AS. (2000). Invited review: Mechanisms of ventilator-induced lung injury: a perspective. *J Appl Physiol.* 89, pp. 1645–1655.

50. Dreyfuss D and Saumon G. (1998). Ventilator-induced lung injury: Lessons from experimental studies. *Am J Respir Crit Care Med.* 157, pp. 294–323.

51. Exley AR, Cohen J, Buurman W, *et al.* (1990). Monoclonal antibody to TNF in severe septic shock. *Lancet.* 335, pp. 1275–1277.

52. Fan E, Brodie D, Slutsky AS. (2018). Acute respiratory distress syndrome: Advances in diagnosis and treatment. *JAMA.* 319(7), pp. 698–710.

53. Fan E, Needham DM, Stewart TE. (2005). Ventilatory management of acute lung injury and acute respiratory distress syndrome. *JAMA.* 294, pp. 2889–2896.

54. Favreau DJ, Meessen-Pinard M, Desforges M, Talbot PJ. (2012). Human coronavirus-induced neuronal programmed cell death is cyclophilin D dependent and potentially caspase dispensable. *J Virol.* 86(1), pp. 81–93.

55. Fink K, Duval A, Martel A, *et al.* (2008). Dual role of NOX2 in respiratory syncytial virus- and sendai virus-induced activation of NF-kappaB in airway epithelial cells. *J Immunol.* 180(10), pp. 6911–6922.

56. Fleming MD, Weigelt JA, Brewer V, McIntire D. (1992). Effect of helium and oxygen on airflow in a narrowed airway. *Arch Surg.* 127, pp. 956– 959.

57. Frank JA, Pittet J-F, Wray C, Matthay MA. (2008). Protection from experimental ventilator-induced acute lung injury by IL-1 receptor blockade. *Thorax.* 63, pp. 147–153.

58. Fukuda K, Asoh S, Ishikawa M, *et al.* (2007). Inhalation of hydrogen gas suppresses hepatic injury caused by ischemia/reperfusion through reducing oxidative stress. *Biochem Biophys Res Commun.* 361(3), pp. 670–674.

59. Fukumoto J, Cox R Jr, Fukumoto I, *et al.* (2016). Deletion of ASK1 protects against hyperoxia-induced acute lung injury. *PLoS One.* 11, pp. e0147652.

60. Fung SY, Yuen KS, Ye ZW, *et al.* (2020). A tug-of-war between severe acute respiratory syndrome coronavirus 2 and host antiviral defence: Lessons from other pathogenic viruses. *Emerg Microbes Infect.* 9(1), pp. 558–570.

61. Fung TS, Liu DX. (2019). Human coronavirus: host-pathogen interaction. *Annu Rev Microbiol.* 73, pp. 529–557.

62. Gao H, Li LY, Zhang M, Zhang Q. (2016). Inactivated Sendai virus induces apoptosis mediated by reactive oxygen species in murine melanoma cells. *Biomed Environ Sci.* 29(12), pp. 877–884

63. Gao L, Jiang D, Geng J, *et al.* (2019). Hydrogen inhalation attenuated bleomycin-induced pulmonary fibrosis by inhibiting transforming growth factor-β1 and relevant oxidative stress and epithelial-to-mesenchymal transition. *Exp Physiol.* 104(12), pp. 1942–1951.

64. Gassen NC, Niemeyer D, Muth D, *et al.* (2019). SKP2 attenuates autophagy through Beclin1-ubiquitination and its inhibition reduces MERS-Coronavirus infection. *Nat Commun.* 10, pp. 5770.

65. Ge L, Yang M, Yang NN, *et al.* (2017). Molecular hydrogen: A preventive and therapeutic medical gas for various diseases. *Oncotarget.* 8(60), pp. 102653–102673.

66. Geto Z, Molla MD, Challa F, *et al.* (2020). Mitochondrial dynamic dysfunction as a main triggering factor for inflammation associated chronic non-communicable diseases. *J Inflamm Res.* 13, pp. 97–107.

67. Ghadiali SN and Gaver DP. (2008). Biomechanics of liquid-epithelium interactions in pulmonary airways. *Respir Physiol Neurobiol.* 163(1–3), pp. 232–243.

68. Gharib B, Hanna S, Abdallahi OM, *et al.* (2001). Anti-inflammatory properties of molecular hydrogen: Investigation on parasite-induced liver inflammation. *C R Acad Sci III.* 324(8), pp. 719–724.

69. Glauser SC, Glauser EM, Rusy BF. (1969). Influence of gas density and viscosity on the work of breathing. *Arch Environ Health*. 19, pp. 654– 660.

70. Go HS, Seo JE, Kim KC, *et al.* (2011). Valproic acid inhibits neural progenitor cell death by activation of NF-κB signaling pathway and up-regulation of Bcl-XL. *J Biomed Sci*. 18(1), pp. 48.

71. Gong X, Zhang L, Jiang R, *et al.* (2013). Antiinflammatory effects of mangiferin on sepsis-induced lung injury in mice via up-regulation of heme oxygenase-1. *J Nutr*. 24, pp. 1173.

72. Gong ZJ, Guan JT, Ren XZ, *et al.* (2016). [Protective effect of hydrogen on the lung of sanitation workers exposed to haze]. *Zhonghua Jie He He Hu Xi Za Zhi*. 39(12), pp. 916–923. (in Chinese)

73. Grandvaux N, Mariani M, Fink K. (2015). Lung epithelial NOX/DUOX and respiratory virus infections. *Clin Sci (Lond)*. 128(6), pp. 337–347.

74. Griffiths LM, Doudican NA, Shadel GS, Doetsch PW. (2009). Mitochondrial DNA oxidative damage and mutagenesis in *Saccharomyces cerevisiae*. *Methods Mol Biol*. 554, pp. 267–286.

75. Gu J, Gong E, Zhang B, *et al.* (2005). Multiple organ infection and the pathogenesis of SARS. *J Exp Med*. 202(3), pp. 415–424.

76. Guan P, Lin XM, Yang SC, *et al.* (2019). Hydrogen gas reduces chronic intermittent hypoxia-induced hypertension by inhibiting sympathetic nerve activity and increasing vasodilator responses via the antioxidation. *J Cell Biochem*. 120(3), pp. 3998–4008.

77. Guan P, Sun ZM, Luo LF, *et al.* (2019). Hydrogen gas alleviates chronic intermittent hypoxia-induced renal injury through reducing iron overload. *Molecules*. 24(6), pp. pii: E1184.

78. Guan P, Sun ZM, Luo LF, *et al.* (2019). Hydrogen protects against chronic intermittent hypoxia induced renal dysfunction by promoting autophagy and alleviating apoptosis. *Life Sci*. 225, pp. 46–54.

79. Guan WJ, Chen RC, Zhong NS (2020). Strategies for the prevention and management of coronavirus disease 2019. *Eur Respir.* (in press).

80. Guan WJ, Wei CH, Zhong NS. (2020). Hydrogen/oxygen mixed gas inhalation improves disease severity and dyspnea in patients with Coronavirus disease 2019 in a recent multicenter, open-label clinical trial. *J Thorac Dis.* 12(6), pp. 3448–3452.

81. Guo YR, Cao QD, Hong ZS, *et al.* (2020). The origin, transmission and clinical therapies on coronavirus disease 2019 (COVID-19) outbreak — an update on the status. *Mil Med Res.* 7(1), pp. 11.

82. Han KY, Kim KT, Joung JG, *et al.* (2018). SIDR: simultaneous isolation and parallel sequencing of genomic DNA and total RNA from single cells. *Genome Res.* 28(1), pp. 75–87.

83. Harijith A, Ebenezer DL, Natarajan V .(2014). Reactive oxygen species at the crossroads of inflammasome and inflammation. *Front Physiol.* 5, pp. 352.

84. He C and Klionsky DJ. (2009). Regulation mechanisms and signaling pathways of autophagy. *Annu Rev Genet.* 43, pp. 67–93.

85. He JH, Tao HY, Yan YM, *et al.* (2020). Molecular mechanism of evolution and human infection with SARS-CoV-2. *Viruses.* 12(4), pp. 428; https://doi.org/10.3390/v12040428. Hennet T, Ziltener HJ, Frei K, Peterhans E. (1992). A kinetic study of immune mediators in the lungs of mice infected with influenza A virus. *J Immunol.* 149(3), pp. 932–939.

86. Hirano SI, Ichikawa Y, Kurokawa R, *et al.* (2020). A "philosophical molecule," hydrogen may overcome senescence and intractable diseases. *Med Gas Res.* 10(1), pp. 47–49.

87. Hoegl S, Bachmann M, Scheiermann P, *et al.* (2011). Protective properties of inhaled IL-22 in a model of ventilator-induced lung injury. *Am J Respir Cell Mol Biol.* 44, pp. 369–376.

88. Hoegl S, Boost KA, Czerwonka H, *et al.* (2009). Inhaled IL-10 reduces biotrauma and mortality in a model of ventilator-induced lung injury. *Respir Med.* 103, pp. 463–470.

89. Hoetzel A, Dolinay T, Vallbracht S, *et al.* (2008). Carbon monoxide protects against ventilator-induced lung injury via PPAR-gamma and inhibition of Egr-1. *Am J Respir Crit Care Med.* 177, pp. 1223–1232.

90. Hong Y, Sun LI, Sun R, *et al.* (2016). Combination therapy of molecular hydrogen and hyperoxia improves survival rate and organ damage in a zymosan-induced generalized inflammation model. *Exp Ther Med.* 11(6), pp. 2590–2596.

91. Hosakote YM, Jantzi PD, Esham DL, *et al.* (2011). Viral-mediated inhibition of antioxidant enzymes contributes to the pathogenesis of severe respiratory syncytial virus bronchiolitis. *Am J Respir Crit Care Med.* 183(11), pp. 1550–1560.

92. Hosakote YM, Liu T, Castro SM, *et al.* (2009). Respiratory syncytial virus induces oxidative stress by modulating antioxidant enzymes. *Am J Respir Cell Mol Biol.* 41(3), pp. 348–357.

93. Huang CL, Wang YM, Li XW, *et al.* (2020). Clinical features of patients infected with 2019 novel coronavirus in Wuhan, China. *Lancet.* 395(10223), pp. 497–506.

94. Huang CS, Kawamura T, Lee S, *et al.* (2010). Hydrogen inhalation ameliorates ventilator-induced lung injury. *Crit Care.* 14(6), pp. R234.

95. Huang CS, Kawamura T, Peng X, *et al.* (2011). Hydrogen inhalation reduced epithelial apoptosis in ventilator-induced lung injury via a mechanism involving nuclear factor-kappa B activation. *Biochem Biophys Res Commun.* 408(2), pp. 253–258.

96. Huang CS, Kawamura T, Toyoda Y, Nakao A. (2010). Recent advances in hydrogen research as a therapeutic medical gas. *Free Rad Res.* 44(9), pp. 971–982.

97. Huang P, Wei S, Huang W, *et al.* (2019). Hydrogen gas inhalation enhances alveolar macrophage phagocytosis in an ovalbumin-induced asthma model. *Int Immunopharmacol.* 74, 105646. doi: 10.1016/j.intimp.2019.05.031.

98. Hussin AR and Byrareddy SN. (2020).The epidemiology and pathogenesis of coronavirus disease (COVID-19) outbreak. *J Autoimmun.* 109, pp. 102433.

99. Iida A, Nosaka N, Yumoto T, *et al.* (2016). The clinical application of hydrogen as a medical treatment. *Acta Med Okayama.* 70(5), pp. 331–337.

100. Imai Y, Kawano T, Iwamoto S, *et al.* (1999). Intratracheal anti-tumor necrosis factor-alpha antibody attenuates ventilator-induced lung injury in rabbits. *J Appl Physiol.* 87, pp. 510–515.

101. Imai Y, Parodo J, Kajikawa O, *et al.* (2003). Injurious mechanical ventilation and end-organ epithelial cell apoptosis and organ dysfunction in an experimental model of acute respiratory distress syndrome. *JAMA.* 289(16), pp. 2104–2112.

102. Ishibashi T. (2019). Therapeutic efficacy of molecular hydrogen: A new mechanistic insight. *Curr Pharm Des.* 25(9), pp. 946–955.

103. Ishihara G, Kawamoto K, Komori N, Ishibashi T. (2019). Molecular hydrogen suppresses superoxide generation in the mitochondrial complex I and reduced mitochondrial membrane potential. *Biochem Biophys Res Commun.* 522(4), pp. 965–970.

104. Jaber S, Carlucci A, Boussarsar M. (2001). Helium-oxygen in the postextubation period decreases inspiratory effort. *Am J Respir Crit Care Med.* 164, pp. 633–637.

105. Janssen YMW, Van Houten B, Borm PJA, Mossman BT. (1993). Biology of disease: Cell and tissue responses to oxidative damage. *Lab Invest.* 69(3), pp. 261–274.

106. Kallet RH and Matthay MA. (2013). Hyperoxic acute lung injury. *Respir Care.* 58(1), pp. 123–141.

107. Kamimura N, Ichimiya H, Iuchi K, Ohta S. (2016). Molecular hydrogen stimulates the gene expression of transcriptional coactivator PGC-1α

to enhance fatty acid metabolism. *NPJ Aging Mech Dis.* 2, pp. 16008.

108. Kamphorst AO, Wieland A, Nasti T, *et al.* (2017). Rescue of exhausted CD8 T cells by PD-1-targeted therapies is CD28-dependent. *Science.* 355(6332), pp. 1423–1427.

109. Kannan S, Shaik Syed Ali P, Sheeza A, Hemalatha K. (2020). COVID-19 (novel coronavirus 2019) — recent trends. *Eur Rev Med Pharmacol Sci.* 24(4), pp. 2006–2011.

110. Kawamura T, Higashida K, Muraoka I. (2020). Application of molecular hydrogen as a novel antioxidant in sports science. *Oxid Med Cell Longev.* 2020, pp. 2328768.

111. Kawamura T, Huang CS, Tochigi N, *et al.* (2010). Inhaled hydrogen gas therapy for prevention of lung transplant-induced ischemia/reperfusion injury in rats. *Transplantation.* 90(12), pp. 1344–1351

112. Kawamura T, Wakabayashi N, Shigemura N, *et al.* (2013). Hydrogen gas reduces hyperoxic lung injury via the Nrf2 pathway in vivo. *Am J Physiol Lung Cell Mol Physiol.* 304(10), pp. L646–656.

113. Kensler TW, Wakabayashi N, Biswal S. (2007). Cell survival responses to environmental stresses via the Keap1-Nrf2-ARE pathway. *Annu Rev Pharmacol Toxicol.* 47, pp. 89–116.

114. Khomich OA, Kochetkov SN, Bartosch B, *et al.* (2018). Redox biology of respiratory viral infections. *Viruses.* 10(8), pp. 392.

115. Kim SI, Kwak JH, Zachariah M, *et al.* (2007). TGF-beta-activated kinase 1 and TAK1-binding protein 1 cooperate to mediate TGF-beta1-induced MKK3-p38 MAPK activation and stimulation of type I collagen. *Am J Physiol Renal Physiol.* 292, pp. F1471–1478.

116. Kindler E, Jónsdóttir HR, Muth D, *et al.* (2013). Efficient replication of the novel human betacoronavirus EMC on primary human epithelium highlights its zoonotic potential. *MBio.* 4, pp. e00611–12.

117. Kohama K, Yamashita H, Aoyama-Ishikawa M, *et al.* (2015). Hydrogen inhalation protects against acute lung injury induced by hemorrhagic shock and resuscitation. *Surgery*. 158(2), pp. 399–407.

118. Krähling V, Stein DA, Spiegel M, *et al.* (2009). Severe acute respiratory syndrome coronavirus triggers apoptosis via protein kinase R but is resistant to its antiviral activity. *J. Virol*. 83(5), pp. 2298–3093.

119. Kress JP and Hall JB. (2014). ICU-acquired weakness and recovery from critical illness. *N Engl J Med*. 371(3), pp. 287–288.

120. Krizbai IA, Bauer H, Bresgen N, *et al.* (2005). Effect of oxidative stress on the junctional proteins of cultured cerebral endothelial cells. *Cell Mol Neurobiol*. 25(1), pp. 129–139.

121. Kumari S, Badana AK, Mohan GM, *et al.* (2018). Reactive oxygen species: A key constituent in cancer survival. *Biomark Insights*. 13, pp. 1177 271918755391.

122. Kwak MK, Itoh K, Yamamoto M, Kensler TW. (2002). Enhanced expression of the transcription factor Nrf2 by cancer chemopreventive agents: role of antioxidant response element-like sequences in the nrf2 promoter. *Mol Cell Biol*. 22(9), pp. 2883–2892.

123. Lake MA. (2020). What we know so far: COVID-19 current clinical knowledge and research. *Clin Med* (Lond). 20(2), pp. 124–127.

124. Law HK, Cheung CY, Ng HY, *et al.* (2005). Chemokine up-regulation in SARS-coronavirus-infected, monocyte-derived human dendritic cells. *Blood*. 106(7), pp. 2366–2374.

125. Lazrak A, Iles KE, Liu G, *et al.* (2009). Influenza virus M2 protein inhibits epithelial sodium channels by increasing reactive oxygen species. *FASEB J*. 23(11), pp. 3829–3842.

126. LeBaron TW, Kura B, Kalocayova B, *et al.* (2019). Hydrogen significantly reduces the effects of oxidative stress. *Molecules*. 24(11), pp. 2076.

127. Lee CH, Chen RF, Liu JW, *et al*. (2004). Altered p38 mitogen-activated protein kinase expression in different leukocytes with increment of immunosuppressive mediators in patients with severe acute respiratory syndrome. *J Immunol*. 172, pp. 7841–7847.

128. Lee JH and Paull TT. (2020). Mitochondria at the crossroads of ATM-mediated stress signaling and regulation of reactive oxygen species. *Redox Biol*. 32, pp. 101511.

129. Levander OA. (1997). Nutrition and newly emerging viral diseases: An overview. *J Nutr*. 127(5), pp. 948S–950S.

130. Levitt MD. (1969). Production and excretion of hydrogen gas in man. *N Engl J Med*. 281(3), pp. 122–127.

131. Levitt MD. (1980). Intestinal gas production--recent advances in flatology. *N Engl J Med*. 302(26), pp. 1474–1475.

132. Li J and Fan JG. (2020). Characteristics and mechanism of liver injury in 2019 coronavirus disease. *J Clin Transl Hepatol*. 8(1), pp. 13–17.

133. Li L, Li X, Zhang Z, Liu L, *et al*. (2020). Protective mechanism and clinical application of hydrogen in myocardial ischemia-reperfusion injury. *Pak J Biol Sci*. 23(2), pp. 103–112.

134. Li PC, Wang BR, Li CC, *et al*. (2018). Seawater inhalation induces acute lung injury via ROS generation and the endoplasmic reticulum stress pathway. *Int J Mol Med*. 41(5), pp. 2505–2516.

135. Li S, *et al*. (2016) 5-Aminolevulinic acid combined with ferrous iron ameliorate ischemia-reperfusion injury in the mouse fatty liver model. *Biochem Biophys Res Commun*. 470, pp. 900–906.

136. Li SW, Fujino M, Ichimaru N, *et al*. (2018). Molecular hydrogen protects against ischemia-reperfusion injury in a mouse fatty liver model via regulating HO-1 and Sirt1 expression. *Sci Rep*. 8, pp. 14019.

137. Li SW, Wang CY, Jou YJ, *et al.* (2016). SARS coronavirus papain-like protease induces Egr-1-dependent up-regulation of TGF-β1 via ROS/ p38 MAPK/STAT3 pathway. *Sci Rep.* 6, pp. 25754.

138. Li W, Yang S, Yu FY, *et al.* (2018). Hydrogen ameliorates chronic intermittent hypoxia-induced neurocognitive impairment via inhibiting oxidative stress. *Brain Res Bull.* 143, pp. 225–233.

139. Li Y, Xie K, Chen H, Wang G, Yu Y. (2015). Hydrogen gas inhibits high-mobility group box 1 release in septic mice by upregulation of heme oxygenase 1. *J Surg Res.* 196(1), pp. 136–148.

140. Li YC, Bai WZ, Hashikawa T. (2020). The neuroinvasive potential of SARS-CoV2 may play a role in the respiratory failure of COVID-19 patients. *J Med Virol.* doi: 10.1002/jmv.25728.

141. Liang C1, Liu X, Liu L, He D. (2012). [Effect of hydrogen inhalation on p38 MAPK activation in rats with lipopolysaccharide- induced acute lung injury]. *Nan Fang Yi Ke Da Xue Xue Bao.* 32(8), pp. 1211–1213. (in Chinese)

142. Lin N, Ji ZQ, Huang CW. (2017). Smad7 alleviates glomerular mesangial cell proliferation via the ROS-NF-κB pathway. *Exp Cell Res.* 361(2), pp. 210–216.

143. Lin X, Wang R, Zou W, *et al.* (2016). The influenza virus H5N1 infection can induce ROS production for viral replication and host cell death in A549 cells modulated by human Cu/Zn superoxide dismutase (SOD1) overexpression. *Viruses.* 8(1), pp. 13.

144. Liu DX, Fung TS, Chong KK-L, *et al.* (2014). Accessory proteins of SARS-CoV and other coronaviruses. *Antiviral Res.* 109, pp. 97–109.

145. Liu G, Yu YH, Xie KL. (2018). [Effect of high concentration of hydrogen gas inhalation on postoperative delirium in elderly patients receiving hip fracture surgery]. *J Clin Anesthesiology.* 34, pp. 5–8. (in Chinese)

146. Liu H, Liang X, Wang D, *et al*. (2015). Combination therapy with nitric oxide and molecular hydrogen in a murine model of acute lung injury. *Shock*. 43(5), pp. 504–511.

147. Liu J, Zheng X, Tong Q, *et al*. (2020). Overlapping and discrete aspects of the pathology and pathogenesis of the emerging human pathogenic coronaviruses SARS-CoV, MERS-CoV, and 2019-nCoV. *J Med Virol*. 92(5), pp. 491–494.

148. Liu W, Shan LP, Dong XS, *et al*. (2013). Combined early fluid resuscitation and hydrogen inhalation attenuates lung and intestine injury. *World J Gastroenterol*. 19(4), pp. 492–502.

149. Liu X, Ma C, Wang X, *et al*. (2017). Hydrogen coadministration slows the development of COPD-like lung disease in a cigarette smoke-induced rat model. *Int J Chron Obstruct Pulmon Dis*. 12, pp. 1309–1324.

150. Liu, Liu Q, Wang RS. (2020). Anatomy report of the corpse system of a new type of coronavirus pneumonia. *Shanghai J Foren Med*. [in Chinese]

151. Lu W, Li D, Hu J, *et al*. (2018). Hydrogen gas inhalation protects against cigarette smoke-induced COPD development in mice. *J Thorac Dis*. 10(6), pp. 3232–3243.

152. Madahar P and Beitler JR. (2020). Emerging concepts in ventilation-induced lung injury. *Version 1*. F1000Res. 9, pp. 222.

153. Martinon F, Pétrilli V, Mayor A, *et al*. (2006). Gout-associated uric acid crystals activate the NALP3 inflammasome. *Nature*. 440(7081), pp. 237–241.

154. Meng X, Xu H, Dang Y, *et al*. (2019). Hyperoxygenated hydrogen-rich solution suppresses lung injury induced by hemorrhagic shock in rats. *J Surg Res*. 239, pp. 103–114.

155. Mittal M, Siddiqui MR, Tran K, *et al*. (2014). Reactive oxygen species in inflammation and tissue injury. *Antioxid Redox Signal*. 20(7), pp. 1126–1167.

156. Moon DH, Kang DY, Haam SJ, *et al*. (2019). Hydrogen gas inhalation ameliorates lung injury after hemorrhagic shock and resuscitation. *J Thorac Dis*. 11(4), pp. 1519–1527.

157. Nakahira K, Haspel JA, Rathinam VA, *et al*. (2011). Autophagy proteins regulate innate immune responses by inhibiting the release of mitochondrial DNA mediated by the NALP3 inflammasome. *Nat Immunol*. 12, pp. 222–230.

158. Nakamura, K. *et al*. (2017). Macrophage heme oxygenase-1-SIRT1-p53 axis regulates sterile inflammation in liver ischemia-reperfusion injury. *J Hepatol*. 67(6), pp. 1232–1242.

159. Nencioni A, Wesselborg S, Brossart P. (2003). Role of peroxisome proliferator-activated receptor gamma and its ligands in the control of immune responses. *Crit Rev Immunol*. 23(1–2), pp. 1–13.

160. Ng CH, Kong SM, Tiong YL, *et al*. (2014). Selective anticancer copper(II)-mixed ligand complexes: targeting of ROS and proteasomes. *Metallomics*. 6(4), pp. 892–906.

161. Nguyen T, Nioi P, Pickett CB.(2009). The Nrf2-antioxidant response element signaling pathway and its activation by oxidative stress. *J Biol Chem*. 284(20), pp. 13291–13295.

162. Nicholls J, Dong XP, Jiang G, Peiris M. (2003). SARS: Clinical virology and pathogenesis. *Respirology*. 8 Suppl, pp. S6–8.

163. Nicholls JM, Poon LL, Lee KC, *et al*. (2003). Lung pathology of fatal severe acute respiratory syndrome. *Lancet*. 361(9371), pp. 1773–1778.

164. Nogueira JE, de Deus JL, Amorim MR, *et al*. (2020). Inhaled molecular hydrogen attenuates intense acute exercise-induced hippocampal inflammation in sedentary rats. *Neurosci Lett*. 715, pp. 134577.

165. Nogueira JE, Passaglia P, Mota CMD, *et al*. (2018). Molecular hydrogen reduces acute exercise-induced inflammatory and oxidative stress status. *Free Radic Biol Med*. 129, pp. 186–193.

166. Ohsawa I, Ishikawa M, Takahashi K, *et al.* (2007). Hydrogen acts as a therapeutic antioxidant by selectively reducing cytotoxic oxygen radicals. *Nat Med.* 13, pp. 688–694.

167. Ohta S. (2014). Molecular hydrogen as a preventive and therapeutic medical gas: Initiation, development and potential of hydrogen medicine. *Pharmacol Ther.* 144(1), pp. 1–11.

168. Opal SM, Fisher CJ, Dhainaut JF, *et al.* (1997). Confirmatory interleukin-1 receptor antagonist trial in severe sepsis: A phase III, randomized, double-blind, placebo-controlled, multicenter trial. The Interleukin-1 Receptor Antagonist Sepsis Investigator Group. *Crit Care Med.* 25, pp. 1115–1124.

169. Pagano A and Brazzazzone-Argiroffo C. (2003). Alveolar cell death in hyperoxia-induced lung injury. *Ann NY Acad Sci.* 1010, pp. 405–416.

170. Palamara AT, Di Francesco P, Ciriolo MR, *et al.* (1996). Cocaine increases Sendai virus replication in cultured epithelial cells: critical role of the intracellular redox status. *Biochem Biophys Res Commun.* 228(2), pp. 579–585.

171. Pendyala S, Natarajan V. (2010). Redox regulation of Nox proteins. *Respir Physiol Neurobiol.* 174(3), pp. 265–271.

172. Perrone LA, Plowden JK, García-Sastre A, *et al.* (2008). H5N1 and 1918 pandemic influenza virus infection results in early and excessive infiltration of macrophages and neutrophils in the lungs of mice. *PLoS Pathog.* 4(8), pp. e1000115.

173. Peterhans E. (1997). Oxidants and antioxidants in viral diseases: Disease mechanisms and metabolic regulation. *J Nutr.* 127(5), pp. 962S–965S.

174. Picca A, Lezza AMS, Leeuwenburgh C, *et al.* (2017). Fueling inflamm-aging through mitochondrial dysfunction: Mechanisms and molecular targets. *Int J Mol Sci.* 18(5), pp. 933.

175. Pilcher JE. (1888). Senn on the diagnosis of gastro-intestinal perforation by the rectal insufflation of hydrogen gas. *Ann Surg.* 8(3), pp. 190–204.

176. Pratt PC. (1958). Pulmonary capillary proliferation induced by O_2 ventilation. *Am J Pathol*. 34(6), pp. 1033–1050.

177. Qian L, Wu Z, Cen J, Pasca S. (2019). Medical application of hydrogen in hematological diseases. *Oxid Med Cell Longev*. 2019, pp. 3917393.

178. Qiu X, Li H, Tang H, *et al*. (2011). Hydrogen inhalation ameliorates lipopolysaccharide-induced acute lung injury in mice. *Int Immunopharmacol*. 11(12), pp. 2130–2137.

179. Ranieri VM, Suter PM, Tortorella C, *et al*. (1999). Effect of mechanical ventilation on inflammatory mediators in patients with acute respiratory distress syndrome: A randomized controlled trial. *JAMA*. 282(1), pp, 54–61.

180. Rogel M. R. *et al*. (2011). Vimentin is sufficient and required for wound repair and remodeling in alveolar epithelial cells. *FASEB J*. 25(1), pp. 3873–3883.

181. Rott R, Klenk H-D, Nagai Y, Tashiro M. (1995). Influenza viruses, cell enzymes, and pathogenicity. *Am J Resp Critl Care Med*. 152(4), pp. S16–S19.

182. Rowlands DJ, Naimul Islam M, Das SR, *et al*. (2011). Activation of TNFR1 ectodomain shedding by mitochondrial Ca^{2+} determines the severity of inflammation in mouse lung microvessels. *J Clin Invest*. 121(5), pp. 1986–1999.

183. Saeidi A, Zandi K, Cheok YY, Saeidi H, *et al*. (2018). T-cell exhaustion in chronic infections: Reversing the state of exhaustion and reinvigorating optimal protective immune responses. *Front Immunol*. 9, pp. 2569.

184. Saitoh T, Fujita N, Jang MH, *et al*. (2008). Loss of the autophagy protein Atg16L1 enhances endotoxin-induced IL-1beta production. *Nature*. 456, pp. 264–268.

185. Sano M, Suzuki M, Homma K, *et al*. (2018). Promising novel therapy with hydrogen gas for emergency and critical care medicine. *Acute Med Surg*. 5(2), pp. 113–118.

186. Sato Y, Kajiyama S, Amano A, *et al.* (2008). Hydrogen-rich pure water prevents superoxide formation in brain slices of vitamin C-depleted SMP30/GNL knockout mice. *Biochem Biophys Res Commun.* 375, pp. 346–350.

187. Scharping NE, Menk, AV1 Moreci RS, *et al.* (2016). The tumor microenvironment represses T cell mitochondrial biogenesis to drive intratumoral T cell metabolic insufficiency and dysfunction. *Immunity.* 45(2), pp. 374–388.

188. Selemidis S, Seow HJ, Broughton BR, *et al.* (2013). Nox1 oxidase suppresses influenza a virus-induced lung inflammation and oxidative stress. *PLoS One.* 8(4), pp. e60792.

189. Shanghai Asclepius Meditec Co., Ltd., Shanghai, China. (2019). Summary of clinical trial of hydrogen and oxygen inhalation for AECOPD 2019.

190. Sies H. (2015). Oxidative stress: A concept in redox biology and medicine. *Redox Biol.* 4, pp. 180–183.

191. Singhal T. (2020).A Review of coronavirus disease-2019 (COVID-19). *Indian J Pediatr.* 87(4), pp. 281–286.

192. Skrinskas GJ, Hyland RH, Hutcheon MA. (1983). Using helium-oxygen mixtures in the manage- ment of acute upper airway obstruction. *Can Med Assoc J.* 128, pp. 555–558.

193. Slutsky AS and Tremblay LN (1998). Multiple system organ failure: Is mechanical ventilation a contributing factor? *Am J Resp Crit Care Med.* 157, pp. 1721–1725.

194. Smits SL, *et al.* (2010). Exacerbated innate host response to SARS-CoV in aged non-human primates. *PLoS Pathog.* 6(2), pp. e1000756.

195. Strocchi A, Ellis CJ, Furne JK, Levitt MD. (1994). Study of constancy of hydrogen-consuming flora of human colon. *Dig Dis Sci.* 39(3), pp. 494–497.

196. Takata M, Abe J, Tanaka H, *et al.* (1997). Intraalveolar expression of tumor necrosis factor-alpha gene during conventional and high-frequency ventilation. *Am J Respir Crit Care Med.* 156, pp. 272–279.

197. Tang W, Pan PF, Huang XQ, *et al.* (2020). [A pathological report of three COVID-19 cases by minimally invasive autopsies]. *Zhonghua Bing Li Xue Za Zhi.* 49(0), pp. E009. (in Chinese)

198. Tao G, Song G, Qin S. (2019). Molecular hydrogen: Current knowledge on mechanism in alleviating free radical damage and diseases. *Acta Biochim Biophys Sin (Shanghai).* 51(12), pp. 1189–1197.

199. Tateda K, Deng JC, Moore TA, *et al.* (2003). Hyperoxia mediates acute lung injury and increased lethality in murine legionella pneumonia: The role of apoptosis. *J Immunol.* 170(8), pp. 4209–4216.

200. Terasaki Y, Ohsawa I, Terasaki M, *et al.* (2011). Hydrogen therapy attenuates irradiation-induced lung damage by reducing oxidative stress. *Am J Physiol Lung Cell Mol Physiol.* 301(4), pp. L415–426.

201. Tian S, Hu W, Niu L, *et al.* (2020). Pulmonary pathology of early-phase 2019 novel coronavirus (COVID-19) pneumonia in two patients with lung cancer. *J Thorac Oncol.* pii: S1556-0864(20)30132-5.

202. Tisoncik JR, Korth MJ, Simmons CP, *et al.* (2012). Into the eye of the cytokine storm. *Microbiol Mol Biol Rev.* 76(1), pp. 16–32.

203. To EE, Broughton BR, Hendricks KS, *et al.* (2014). Influenza A virus and TLR7 activation potentiate NOX2 oxidase-dependent ROS production in macrophages. *Free Radic Res.* 48(8), pp. 940–947.

204. Tolle LB, Standiford TJ. (2013). Danger-associated molecular patterns (DAMPs) in acute lung injury. *J Pathol.* 229(2), pp. 145–156.

205. Tremblay LN, Slutsky AS. (1998). Ventilator-induced injury: From barotrauma to biotrauma. *Proc Assoc Am Physicians.* 110, pp. 482–488.

206. Tremblay LN, Slutsky AS. (2006). Ventilator-induced lung injury: From the bench to the bedside. *Intensive Care Med.* 32, pp. 24–33.

207. Tse GM, To KF, Chan PK, *et al.* (2004). Pulmonary pathological features in coronavirus associated severe acute respiratory syndrome (SARS). *J Clin Pathol.* 57, pp. 260–265.

208. Turrens JF. (2003). Mitochondrial formation of reactive oxygen species. *J Physiol.* 552, pp. 335–344.

209. Unger BL, Ganesan S, Comstock AT, *et al.* (2014). Nod-like receptor X-1 is required for rhinovirus-induced barrier dysfunction in airway epithelial cells. *J Virol.* 88(7), pp. 3705–3718.

210. van der Veen TA, de Groot LES, Melgert BN. (2020). The different faces of the macrophage in asthma. *Curr Opin Pulm Med.* 26(1), pp. 62–68.

211. Venditti P, Di Meo S. [2020]. The role of reactive oxygen species in the life cycle of the mitochondrion. *Int J Mol Sci.* 21(6), pp. E2173.

212. Vlahos R, Stambas J, Selemidis S. (2012). Suppressing production of reactive oxygen species (ROS) for influenza A virus therapy. *Trends Pharmacol Sci.* 33, pp. 3–8.

213. Vyas-Read S, Wang W, Kato S, *et al.* (2014). Hyperoxia induces alveolar epithelial-to-mesenchymal cell transition. *Am J Physiol Lung Cell Mol Physiol.* 306(4), pp. L326–340.

214. Wang P, Zhao M, Chen Z, *et al.* (2020). Hydrogen gas attenuates hypoxic-ischemic brain injury via regulation of the MAPK/HO-1/PGC-1a pathway in neonatal rats. *Oxid Med Cell Longev.* 2020, pp. 6978784.

215. Weinberg SE, Sena LA, Chandel NS. (2015). Mitochondria in the regulation of innate and adaptive immunity. *Immunity.* 42(3), pp. 406–417.

216. Wherry EJ, Ha SJ, Kaech SM, *et al.* (2007). Molecular signature of CD8+ T cell exhaustion during chronic viral infection. *Immunity.* 27(4), pp. 670–684.

217. Wilson MR, Choudhury S, Takata M. (2005). Pulmonary inflammation induced by high-stretch ventilation is mediated by tumor necrosis

factor signaling in mice. *Am J Physiol Lung Cell Mol Physiol.* 288, pp. L599–607.

218. Wong CK, Lam CW, Wu AK, *et al.* (2004). Plasma inflammatory cytokines and chemokines in severe acute respiratory syndrome. *Clin Exp Immunol.* 136(1), pp. 95–103.

219. Woodfin A, Voisin MB, Nourshargh S. (2010). Recent developments and complexities in neutrophil transmigration. *Curr Opin Hematol.* 17, pp. 9–17.

220. Xie K, Yu Y, Huang Y, *et al.* (2012). Molecular hydrogen ameliorates lipopolysaccharide-induced acute lung injury in mice through reducing inflammation and apoptosis. *Shock.* 37(5), pp. 548–555.

221. Xie K, Yu Y, Pei Y, *et al.* (2010). Protective effects of hydrogen gas on murine polymicrobial sepsis via reducing oxidative stress and HMGB1 release. *Shock.* 34, pp. 90–97.

222. Xiong Y, Liu Y, Cao L, *et al.* (2020). Transcriptomic characteristics of bronchoalveolar lavage fluid and peripheral blood mononuclear cells in COVID-19 patients. *Emerg Microbes Infect. 9(1), pp. 761–770.*

223. Xu KC and Chen JB. (2020). *Clinical Hydrogen Oncology.* Singapore: World Scientific (in press).

224. Xu Z, Shi L, Wang YJ, *et al.* (2020). Pathological findings of COVID-19 associated with acute respiratory distress syndrome. *Lancet Respir Med.* https:// pubmed.ncbi. nlm. nih.gov/32085846.

225. Yang N and Shen HM. (2020). Targeting the endocytic pathway and autophagy process as a novel therapeutic strategy in COVID-19. *Int J Biol Sci.* 16(10), pp. 1724–1731.

226. Yang Q, Liu X, Yao Z, *et al.* (2014). Penehyclidine hydrochloride inhibits the release of high-mobility group box 1 in lipopolysaccharide-

activated RAW264.7 cells and cecal ligation and puncture-induced septic mice. *J Surg Res.* 186, pp. 310.

227. Yao W, Guo A, Han X, *et al*. (2019). Aerosol inhalation of a hydrogen-rich solution restored septic renal function. *Aging* (*Albany NY*). 11(24), pp. 12097–12113.

228. Ye S, Lowther S, Stambas J. (2015). Inhibition of reactive oxygen species production ameliorates inflammation induced by influenza A viruses via upregulation of SOCS1 and SOCS3. *J Virol.* 89(5), pp. 2672–2683.

229. Ying Y, Xu H, Yao M, Qin Z. (2017). Protective effect of hydrogen-saturated saline on acute lung injury induced by oleic acid in rats. *J Orthop Surg Res.* 12(1), pp. 134.

230. Yu Y, Yang YY, Yang M, *et al*. (2019). Hydrogen gas reduces HMGB1 release in lung tissues of septic mice in an Nrf2/HO-1-dependent pathway. *Intern Immunopharmacol.* 69, pp. 11–18.

231. Zhang H, Liu L, Yu Y, *et al*. (2016).[Role of Rho/ROCK signaling pathway in the protective effects of hydrogen against acute lung injury in septic mice]. *Zhonghua Wei Zhong Bing Ji Jiu Yi Xue.* 28(5), pp. 40–406. (in Chinese)

232. Zhang HL, Liu YF, Luo XR, *et al*. (2011). Saturated hydrogen saline protects rats from acute lung injury induced by paraquat. *World J Emerg Med.* 2(2), pp. 149–153.

233. Zhang J, Zhou H, Liu J, *et al*. (2019). Protective effects of hydrogen inhalation during the warm ischemia phase against lung ischemia-reperfusion injury in rat donors after cardiac death. *Microvasc Res.* 125, pp. 103885.

234. Zhang N, Deng CW, Zhang XX, *et al*. (2018). Inhalation of hydrogen gas attenuates airway inflammation and oxidative stress in allergic asthmatic mice. *Asthma Res Pract.* 4, pp. 3.

235. Zhang ZY, Fang YJ, Luo YJ, *et al*. (2019). The role of medical gas in stroke: An updated review. *Med Gas Res*. 9(4), pp. 221–228.

236. Zhao YS, An JR, Yang S, *et al*. (2019). Hydrogen and oxygen mixture to improve cardiac dysfunction and myocardial pathological changes induced by intermittent hypoxia in rats. *Oxid Med Cell Longev*. 2019, pp. 7415212.

237. Zhong NS, Zheng ZG, Sun WZ, *et al*. (2020). Hydrogen/oxygen therapy is superior to oxygen therapy for the treatment an acute exacerbation of chronic obstructive pulmonary disease: results of a multicenter, randomized, double-blind, parallel-group controlled trial (in press).

238. Zhou R, Tardivel A, Thorens B, *et al*. (2010). Thioredoxin-interacting protein links oxidative stress to inflammasome activation. *Nat Immunol*. 11(2), pp. 136–140.

239. Zhou ZQ, Zhong CH, Su ZQ, *et al*. (2018). Breathing hydrogen-oxygen mixture decreases inspiratory effort in patients with tracheal stenosis. *Clin Invest*. doi: 1159/ 000492031.

240. Zhu C, Wang X, Huang Z, *et al*. (2007). Apoptosis-inducing factor is a major contributor to neuronal loss induced by neonatal cerebral hypoxia-ischemia. *Cell Death Differ*. 14(4), pp. 775–784.

241. Zhu N, Zhang D, Wang W, *et al*. (2020). A novel coronavirus from patients with pneumonia in China, 2019. *N Engl J Med*. 382(8), pp. 727–733.

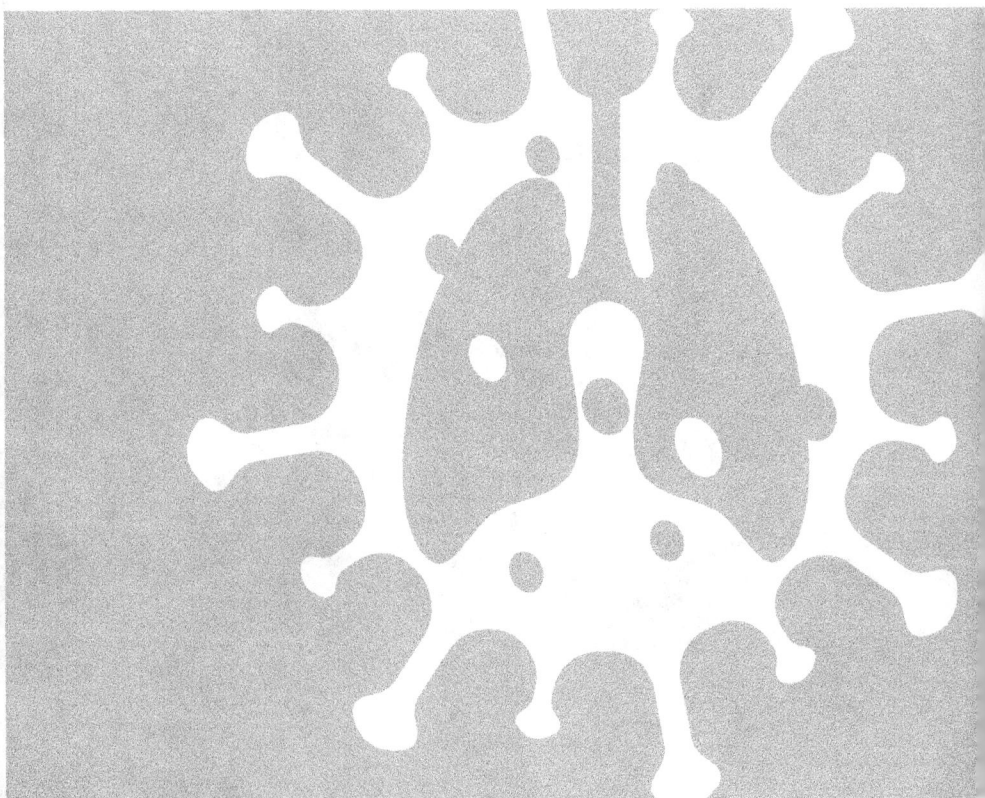

Further Reading

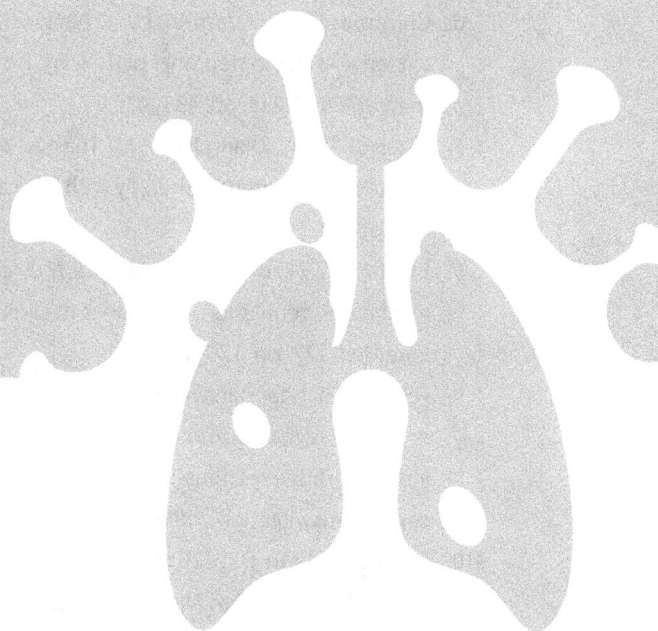

1. Abraini JH, Gardette-Chauffour MC, Martinez E, *et al.* (1994). Psychophysiological reactions in humans during an open sea dive to 500 m with a hydrogen-helium-oxygen mixture. *J Appl Physiol.* 76(3), pp. 1113–1118.

2. Amato MB, Barbas CS, Medeiros DM, *et al.* (1998). Effect of a protective-ventilation strategy on mortality in the acute respiratory distress syndrome. *N Engl J Med.* 338, pp. 347–354.

3. Arbour N, Day R, Newcombe J, Talbot PJ. (2000). Neuroinvasion by human respiratory coronaviruses. *J Virol.* 74(19), pp. 8913–8921.

4. Bem RA, van Woensel JB, Bos AP, *et al.* (2009). Mechanical ventilation enhances lung inflammation and caspase activity in a model of mouse pneumovirus infection. *Am J Physiol Lung Cell Mol Physiol.* 296, pp. L46–56.

5. Boorstein JM, Boorstein SM, Humphries GN, Johnston CC. (1989). Using helium-oxygen mixtures in the emergency management of acute upper airway obstruction. *Ann Emerg Med.* 18, pp. 688–690.

6. Chinopoulos C, Adam-Vizi V. (2006). Calcium, mitochondria and oxidative stress in neuronal pathology. Novel aspects of an enduring theme. *FEBS J.* 273, pp. 433–450.

7. Dixon BJ, Tang J, Zhang JH. (2013). The evolution of molecular hydrogen: A noteworthy potential therapy with clinical significance. *Med Gas Res.* 3(1), pp. 10.

8. Esteban A, Ferguson ND, Meade MO, *et al.* (2008). Evolution of mechanical ventilation in response to clinical research. *Am J Respir Crit Care Med.* 177, pp. 170–177.

9. Fehr AR, Channappanavar R, Jankevicius G, *et al.* (2016). The conserved coronavirus macrodomain promotes virulence and suppresses the innate immune response during severe acute respiratory syndrome coronavirus infection. *mBio.* 7(6), pp. e01721–16.

10. Fung S and Liu DX. (2019). Human coronavirus: Host-pathogen interaction. *Annu. Rev. Microbiol.* 7, pp. 529–557.

11. Furukawa S, Fujita T, Shimabukuro M, *et al.* (2004). Increased oxidative stress in obesity and its impact on metabolic syndrome. *J Clin Invest.* 114, pp. 1752–1761.

12. Gu J, Korteweg C. (2007). Pathology and pathogenesis of severe acute respiratory syndrome. *Am J Pathol.* 170, pp. 1136–1147.

13. Hayashida K, Sano M, Ohsawa I, *et al.* (2008). Inhalation of hydrogen gas reduces infarct size in the rat model of myocardial ischemia-reperfusion injury. *Biochem Biophys Res Commun.* 373, pp. 30–35.

14. He L, Ding Y, Zhang Q, *et al.* (2006). Expression of elevated levels of pro-inflammatory cytokines in SARS-CoV-infected ACE2+ cells in SARS patients: relation to the acute lung injury and pathogenesis of SARS. *J Pathol.* 210(3), pp. 288–297.

15. Hillman NH, Moss TJ, Kallapur SG, *et al.* (2007). Brief, large tidal volume ventilation initiates lung injury and a systemic response in fetal sheep. *Am J Respir Crit Care Med.* 176, pp. 575–581.

16. Hong Y., Chen S., Zhang J. M. (2010). Hydrogen as a selective antioxidant: A review of clinical and experimental studies. *J Intern Medl Res.* 38(6), pp. 1893–1903.

17. Ichihara M, Sobue S, Ito M, Ito M, *et al.* (2015). Beneficial biological effects and the underlying mechanisms of molecular hydrogen — comprehensive review of 321 original articles. *Medical Gas Res.* 5(1), doi: 10.1186/s13618-015-0035-1.

18. Ishihara G, Kawamoto K, Komori N, *et al.* (2020). Molecular hydrogen suppresses superoxide generation in the mitochondrial complex I and reduced mitochondrial membrane potential. *Biochem Biophys Res Commun.* 522(4), pp. 965–970.

19. Ji X, Zheng W, Yao W. (2019). Protective role of hydrogen gas on oxidative damage and apoptosis in intestinal porcine epithelial cells (IPEC-J2) induced by deoxynivalenol: A preliminary study. Toxins (Basel). 12(1), pii: E5.

20. Katira BH. (2019). Ventilator-induced lung injury: Classic and novel concepts. *Respir Care*. 64(6), pp. 629–637.

21. Krynytska IY, Marushchak MI. (2018). The indices of nitrogen (II) oxide system in experimental hepatopulmonary syndrome. *Ukr Biochem J*. 90(5), pp. 91–97.

22. Marshall JC, Cook DJ, Christou NV, *et al*. (1995). Multiple organ dysfunction score: A reliable descriptor of a complex clinical outcome. *Crit Care Med*. 23(10), pp. 1638–1652.

23. Marushchak M, Krynytska I, Petrenko N, Klishch I. (2016). The determination of correlation linkages between level of reactive oxygen species, contents of neutrophils and blood gas composition in experimental acute lung injury. *Georgian Med News*. 4(253), pp. 98–103.

24. Marushchak M, Maksiv K, Krynytska I, *et al*. (2019). The severity of oxidative stress in comorbid chronic obstructive pulmonary disease (COPD) and hypertension: Does it depend on ACE and AGT gene polymorphisms? *J Med Life*. 12(4), pp. 426–434.

25. Matei N, Camara R, Zhang JH. (2018). Emerging mechanisms and novel applications of hydrogen gas therapy. *Med Gas Res*. 8(3), pp. 98–102.

26. Nagata K, Nakashima-Kamimura N, Mikami T, *et al*. (2009). Consumption of molecular hydrogen prevents the stress-induced impairments in hippocampus-dependent learning tasks during chronic physical restraint in mice. *Neuropsychopharmacol*. 34, pp. 501–508.

27. Rahman NA, Fruchter O, Shitrit D, *et al*. (2010). Flexible bronchoscopic management of benign tracheal stenosis: Long term follow-up of 115 patients. *J Cardiothorac Surg*. 5, pp. 2.

28. Schofield JH, Schafer ZT. (2020). Mitochondrial ROS and mitophagy: A complex and nuanced relationship. Antioxid Redox Signal. doi: 10.1089/ars.2020.8058.

29. Silva PL, Negrini D, Rocco PR. (2015). Mechanisms of ventilator-induced lung injury in healthy lungs. *Best Pract Res Clin Anaesthesiol.* 29, pp. 301–313.

30. Sobue S, Yamai K, Ito M, *et al.* (2015). Simultaneous oral and inhalational intake of molecular hydrogen additively suppresses signaling pathways in rodents. *Mol Cell Biochem.* 403, pp. 231–241.

31. Thornton RH, Gordon RL, Kerlan RK, *et al.* (2006). Outcomes of tracheobronchial stent placement for benign disease. *Radiology.* 240, pp. 273–282.

32. Turtle L. (2020). Respiratory failure alone does not suggest central nervous system invasion by SARS-CoV-2. *J Med Virol.* 2020, doi: 10.1002/jmv.25728.

33. van der Staay M, Chatburn RL. (2018). Advanced modes of mechanical ventilation and optimal targeting schemes. *Intensive Care Med Exp.* 6, pp. 30.

34. Vlahos R, Stambas J, Bozinovski S, *et al.* (2011). Inhibition of Nox2 oxidase activity ameliorates influenza A virus-induced lung inflammation. *PLoS Pathog.* 7(2), pp. e1001271

35. Wiegman CH, Michaeloudes C, Haji G, *et al.* (2015). Oxidative stress-induced mitochondrial dysfunction drives inflammation and airway smooth muscle remodeling in patients with chronic obstructive pulmonary disease. *J Allergy Clin Immunol.* 136(3), pp. 769–780.

36. Xu KC, Chen JB. (in press). *Clinical Hydrogen Oncology.* Singapore: World Scientific.

37. Zhilyaev SY, Moskvin AN, Platonova TF, *et al.* (2003). Hyperoxic vasoconstriction in the brain is mediated by inactivation of nitric oxide by superoxide anions. *Neurosci Behav Physiol.* 33(8), pp. 783–787.

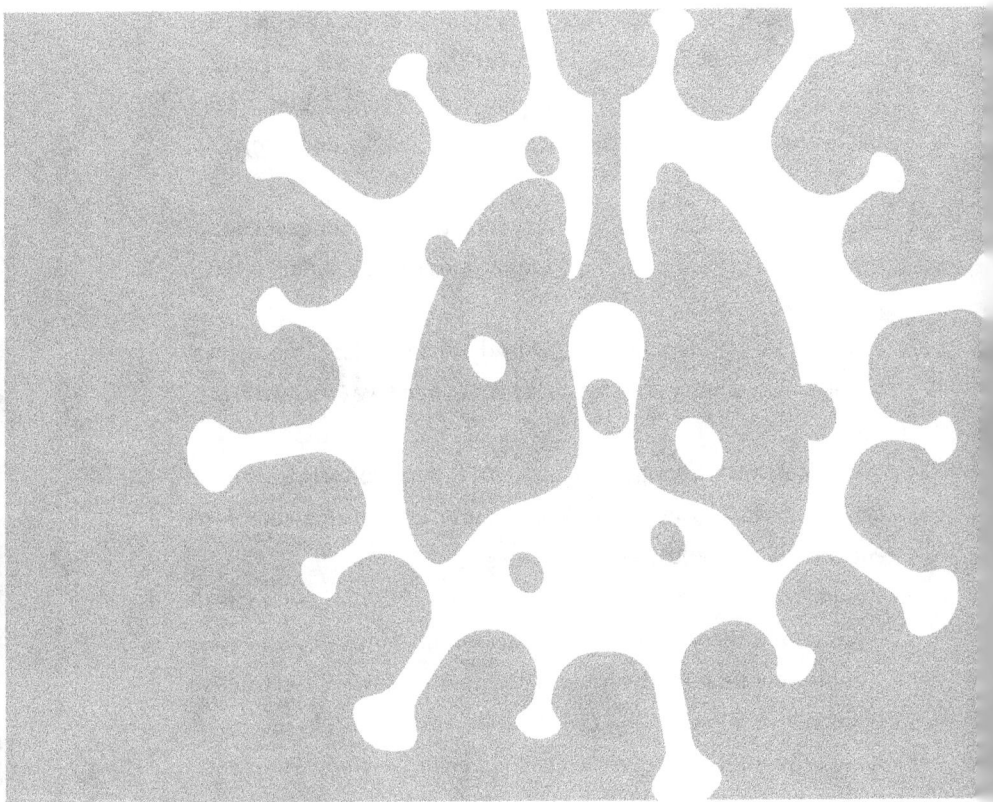

Index

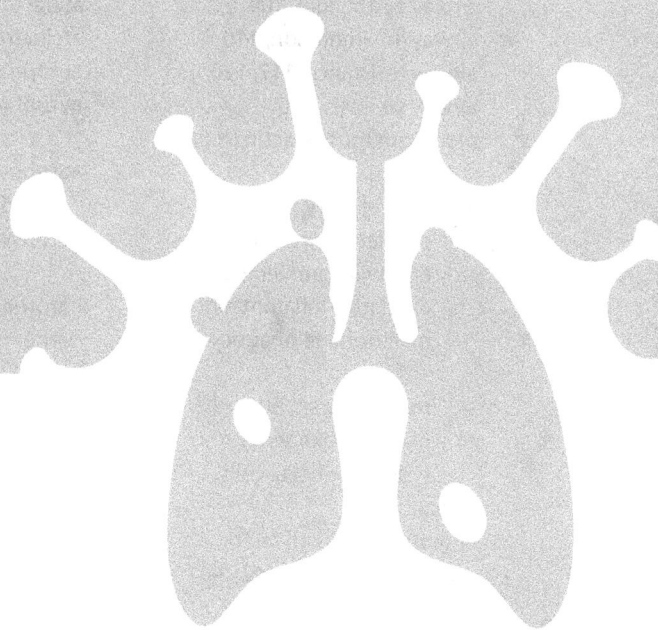